AGE WITH SPIRIT

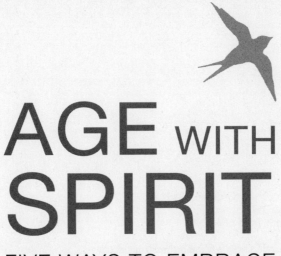

AGE WITH
SPIRIT

FIVE WAYS TO EMBRACE
CHANGE IN YOUR LIFE

Swami Ambikananda Saraswati

Edited by Bri. Manisha Wilmette Brown

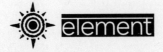

Element
An Imprint of HarperCollins*Publishers*
77–85 Fulham Palace Road
Hammersmith, London W6 8JB

The website address is: www.thorsonselement.com

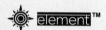

and *Element* are trademarks of
HarperCollins*Publishers* Limited

Published by Element 2003

10 9 8 7 6 5 4 3 2 1

© Swami Ambikananda Saraswati 2003

Swami Ambikananda Saraswati asserts the moral right to
be identified as the author of this work

Text illustrations by Joan Corlass
Illustrations p.193 by PCA Creative

A catalogue record of this book
is available from the British Library

ISBN 0 00 712824 X

Printed and bound in Great Britain by
Creative Print and Design (Wales), Ebbw Vale

Dedicated to

shikara priya
the beloved of the summit

Contents

The Fifth Wave

Acknowledgments

I thank all those who have walked beyond the age where I am now and left their wisdom for me to see. There are many philosophers, writers, artists, and scientists that have challenged me to re-evaluate my vision of myself and of the world. Particularly I thank my beloved guru, Swami Venkatesananda, who always encouraged me to look beyond the most immediate horizon, and Swami Krishnananda, who encouraged me to walk towards that horizon, and Lyall Watson, Richard Leakey, and John Gribbin for showing me new ones.

I also thank Bri. Manisha Wilmette Brown for her conscientious and creative editing and her encouragement when I wanted to give up, and Br. Uddhava Samman for the thousand ways he helps to make my load easier. I thank my friends, students, and patients for letting me use their stories in this book, especially Diederick Reineke, who shared with me the views of anthroposophy on the aging process.

I also thank all at Thorsons, Belinda Budge, Susanna Abbott, Kate Latham, and Lizzie Hutchins in particular, who kept believing in all the possibilities of the project.

Introduction

When I was a child, I spoke as a child, I understood as a child;
But when I became a man I put away childish things.
For now we see through a glass darkly; but then face to face:
then I shall know even as also I am known.

I CORINTHIANS 13:11–12

As a human family, we have reached a time when we are aging in greater numbers than ever before. We are also increasingly questioning the value of any philosophy that separates the spirit from the body. It is a schism that has cut a deep wound in our wholeness and continues to separate us not only from each other but also from ourselves.

I have therefore constructed the "spiritual" practices in this book around a different philosophy – one that calls us to work with our body and our mind in order to reconnect and re-identify with an ageless and timeless self that holds within it our evolving human perfection. In this philosophy, our practices serve to heal the wound of separation by putting the body and mind at the service of a spirit that has always been in the service of our lives. So we may come to experience the presence of something beyond our everyday awareness both with the senses of the body and the understanding of the mind.

Such practices cannot remain confined to a few precious and isolated moments in our lives; they must be integrated into the whole of it. Working in this way with the body – observing and acknowledging its awesome capacities, intelligence, and grace – brings us face to face with our true nature, with a truer self that is less visible to us in youth. As the body recedes in age, its wonder becomes more visible and the spirit that is its source shines through it more clearly.

The spiritual quest of aging, then, is to gather up the courage we have built over the many years we have lived and use it to see better both ourselves and that which we consider "other." Such aging can not only bring the personal rewards of a healthier or even a longer life and expanded consciousness, but also the possibility of a transformation for all of humanity as we become known to ourselves and to each other.

Chapter 1

The Emerging Self

A new voyage has begun for our human family and those of us now aging are its pioneers, exploring a little-known horizon. For the very first time in history we are living past youth and adulthood and continuing on into "old" age in vast numbers. Across the globe 20 years have been added to the average human lifespan, and changes in lifestyle, science, and medicine have nearly doubled the life expectancy in wealthier, industrialized countries. Living to be nearly 100 will soon no longer be the exception, the genetic gift of a few, but the norm.

We, the aging, are the generations that were inoculated and so did not succumb to childhood diseases like polio and smallpox. We are the mothers who could be confident of surviving childbirth ourselves and who knew that our children would also more than likely survive. Added to this, the arrival of antibiotics meant we were not killed off prematurely by infection. Indeed, we have overcome all of these potential killers to live past middle age with the possibility of discovering who we really are and all that we are capable of.

As this is the first time in our history that we are collectively exploring what it is like to be long-lived, we not only need guidance from those already ahead of us, we ourselves must also become the map-makers. It is an exciting challenge – and if we can rise to it, a spiritual adventure awaits us. It may well be, as one old and venerable monk put it, that this is the next step of human evolution – a step in consciousness and self-awareness.

The idea that we are evolving an extended lifespan in order to discover new facets of our human embodiment turns aging from being nothing more than a process of slow dying into an opportunity for self-renewal and discovery. And just as our ancestors had to develop the right musculature to stand upright and view their horizon in a completely new way, so we now need to age in order to know the whole of ourselves and stand fully conscious in the light of that within us which is eternal.

Our collective aging is also a harbinger of great social change. Falling birth rates in most industrialized countries means that people who are over 85 have become the fastest-growing segment of the population. Globally, 1 in 10 people is now over 60 years of age and by 2050 that figure will have risen to 1 in 5. According to Prof. Tom Kirkwood, Head of Gerontology (the science that studies aging) at Newcastle University in England, this offers the potential to change the whole of society by "tipping the balance of power to favour the aged."[1]

All this means that a great many minds have turned their attention to the question of aging. However, instead of being celebrated, this latest triumph of humanity is presented as a "problem": What is to be done with the aging population? We, the aging, must remind ourselves that the problem which aging poses for youth is not a problem for us.

Those of us now beginning to age are the baby boomer generation, the generation that created the social changes of the sixties and that never allowed others to define who we are. Let us bring this energy to our aging. We must explore it as we live it, questioning every theory and challenging every myth – even the ones we ourselves hold dear. And perhaps the myths we are most attached to are the ones we have created about ourselves – who we are and what direction our aging will take.

To take hold of this new power we must first of all become conscious of it and conscious of ourselves. Unlike puberty, when the changes we experience may overwhelm us, by the time we reach middle age we are not only rich in experience, we are also resilient. Therefore, conscious aging – taking full control of the voyage and of our power – becomes a real possibility.

The Mysterious Self

The consciousness of the continuity of our personality continues through the various vicissitudes and changes of life – proving that consciousness itself is changeless.

SWAMI KRISHNANANDA[2]

I have become middle-aged. I only became aware of this when I accidentally caught sight of myself in a store mirror and for just a second did not recognize the woman looking back at me. I was completely stunned. How could I be middle-aged – I had only just begun!

Age suddenly took on a new significance. I began to watch oth-er older people with interest. If there were secrets to aging – and to defying its negative consequences – I meant to uncover them.

That is what I meant to do. But the extraordinary women and men from whom I learned taught me something else. Time and again as I spoke to older people about aging I heard this refrain: "I know I'm 75, but really inside I feel the same as I did at 25."

One delightfully eccentric 92-year-old pinned me down with her steely bright eyes and added, "In fact, you know, I think I felt 25 when I was 5."

So my question became: Who is this 25-year-old, this timeless self that those who age successfully seem to know so intimately? Who is this mysterious presence, situated at an unchanging age of resilience, insight, and personal power, this "self" who witnesses the passage of time in our bodies and minds while remaining true to a rhythm that is quite different from the relentless ticking of the clock?

Those people who continue to grow – rather than merely age – seem to be intimately in touch with this eternally present self. In fact, the older and more aware of their own power they become, the more they identify with this inner self and its purpose – and at times are almost amused by the identity tags of age, appearance, and occupation that society labels us with and that we set so much store by when we are young.

Perhaps the many urgent things we have to do in youth and adulthood – finding the right partner, the right job, creating a family, providing for them, and so on – hide this "self" from our field of vision. It is possible that we have to change through the process of aging in order to experience that which is changeless within.

The Unchanging Supreme reveals Itself through
the constantly changing universe.

THE CHANDOGYA UPANISHAD 17[3]

Looking Forward

All around us there are people who are passing into middle and old age and evolving into the wise. We need to honor their stories because they are walking the path that we will walk.

I have a Yoga student who at 79 came to me after class one day to tell me her news. All the while she held my hand in a firm grip and ended by saying, "I'm having the time of my life." As I looked into her sparkling blue eyes and felt the energy flowing from her hand to mine, I had no reason to disbelieve her. Edna had just been awarded the PhD she had been working on for the past seven years and was about to take a trip to Alaska with her 82-year-old husband as a celebration. It would seem that people like Edna are deeply aware that while the body ages there is an essence that remains forever the same, and as they age they engage with the world from that essence.

That is not to discount the body or to make it seem secondary or unimportant. Quite the contrary, that inner self seems to re-create and drive the body forward, taking us to new places and down unexpected roads. This essence is relentless in its quest to learn and experience, and the body appears to be both a precious means of doing so and a powerful teacher in its own right. By connecting to the inner essence, to the forever 25-year-old within, we begin to understand aging as a journey forward rather than mournfully looking back at youth, which can never be recaptured.

What Edna and people like her have discovered is a way of making that inner eternal being part of their bodily experience, so that they continue to grow as they age. Their knowledge of the inner self, the immortal spirit within, becomes an *embodied* knowing; the practices and habits that are a routine part of daily life – and appear to be of the body – are in fact guided by their spirit. They do not have to force themselves into changing negative habits – their whole lifestyle alters willingly to suit the workings of the inner self. And they bring to this adventure the kind of courage and resourcefulness that only comes with years. They defy the myths of aging that have gathered so much weight they appear as truth, and they live lives that truly reflect the radiance of that unchanging self within.

There is an ancient legend from India called *The Uddhava Gita*, "The Song of Uddhava." A song is different from speech; it requires that we change the pitch of our voice and go beyond our ordinary framework, references, and guides to find not the individual episodes that make up our life, but the poem, the legend, of our life. In "The Song of Uddhava" the aging disciple Uddhava is engaged in dialogue with the great avatar Krishna, an embodiment of the pure unbound spirit. Krishna is about to die, to return to the freedom of the spirit unfettered by flesh and bone, and Uddhava wants to go with him. Krishna denies his disciple this request and Uddhava begs for one last teaching. Krishna's answer is simple and beautiful: "Abandon all that you now think you know about yourself and the world, and explore what you do not know."

> Roam this world free:
> … Whatever you see, hear or touch –
> Know that you do not know it
> For what it is.

THE UDDHAVA GITA 2:6[4]

If we are to discover the hidden power of aging and learn the skills of guiding its emotional and physiological processes, we have to challenge all that we now "know" about it – and about ourselves – and be prepared to explore the unknown.

In doing this we lose our attachment to who we *think* we are and move closer to who we *really* are. And if there is magic in aging, it is that this self within, which the great masters, prophets, and seers of all religions and spiritual paths point us toward, but which is so hard to penetrate in youth, reveals itself naturally and with an easy grace as we grow older and mature.

It is a self that we must finally make our first consideration. Edna had begun studying for her MA degree at the age of 65. She had wanted to continue at university when she completed her first degree but instead, like many other women, she left her studies and turned her attention to her new husband and family. In her early sixties she had nursed her only daughter, who was dying of cancer. After her daughter's death she became determined to make something of the years left to her – to live the old age that had been denied to her child. She reconnected to her spirit – to her eternal 25-year-old self within – and embarked on a journey of fulfillment that she had abandoned in her youth. Her body and mind quickly took direction from this inner self and made themselves available for its purposes.

Like Edna, we need to attune our hearing to a different voice, a voice that speaks from within, the voice of the spirit.

The Return to Wholeness

There is a bridge between now and Infinity
And this bridge is the human spirit ...
When this bridge is crossed even the blind can see;
All sorrow ends and all wounds are healed.

THE CHANDOGYA UPANISHAD 8:4:1 AND 2[5]

We the aging are being called to evolve into a community of shamans to better serve the purpose of the spirit. The shaman is the pivot between heaven and Earth, the conduit through which higher consciousness communicates with everyday consciousness. The mind of the shaman flows like the stream and bends like the reed in the wind to catch the rapture of the spirit and pass it on to the community. Our aging is calling us to such fluidity, to such a challenge of our rigidities, so that the spirit within and without may be more clearly seen by all.

We are rarely and poorly educated about the spirit as something that can unite humanity and heal our personal fragmentation, giving us purpose and direction. In this absence of spirit the body has become the only place where we can pursue immortality, and youth has become the Holy Grail. When we study our history it is of humans struggling and dying but never of humans embodying more than mortality. As we age we thus find ourselves in the position of having to go in search of something which has been denied all our lives. Tragically, each time our search discloses even a glimpse of the spirit, we also see the effects of hiding it: the killing fields of humanity everywhere which could not exist in a world where all flesh is seen as a continuum of the spirit.

We must come to see our wrinkled faces and our changing bodies not as a loss of youth, but as an embodiment of a new human experience in which the spirit has more fully emerged to draw humanity towards its wholeness and interdependence and thus away from the killing fields.

Given that we have reached a time when the weapons we have at our disposal have the capability of destroying all life on this planet, perhaps the very future of humanity lies in the hands of the wise aged as much as it does in those of the new and younger generation.

Spirituality is much more the imperative of age than of youth, and if we embrace the emergence of our spirituality as we age, the social changes which can draw humanity away from the killing fields is in our charge. In Western developed countries we have grown up with an artificial separation of body and spirit for so long that it has taken on the appearance of a universal truth. This separation arose when a great late Renaissance thinker, René Descartes, a deeply religious man, sought a way for scientific endeavor to go ahead without challenging the authority of the Church, which at the time suppressed any such investigation. Descartes was obsessed with knowledge and with how we could "know" anything. From this arose a philosophical formula that separated body and soul so that science could have the body/matter for investigation and the Church could have the mind or soul (mind and soul were not strictly differentiated). This separation saved the lives of many extraordinary scientists of the day and also allowed the inquiry into the body freedom from the restrictions of the Church, thereby contributing to a considerable leap forward in science and medicine. However, we have also suffered as a result of it, for whenever we turn our attention to spiritual inquiry it is seen as having nothing to do with the body. But the experience of spirituality and of aging – and indeed of everything else – *is impossible without the body*.

India never experienced a political or religious climate in which an artificial separation between body and spirit was mandated in the way it has been in Western culture. Philosophical and religious dialogue discussed duality, multiplicity, and oneness in many forms.

One such philosophical viewpoint, called Advaita (meaning "not two") adheres to a universal principle of oneness. It calls us not to some kind of higher knowledge that only a smart few can aspire to, but to the *experience* of ourselves as an integrated whole – as One with everything else included in that One. "Part" in this context is not meant to indicate something fragmented and incomplete, but rather a 'part' that makes the whole complete. In this philosophy, the body, all bodies – animate and inanimate – are part of a supreme and infinite consciousness. And the *appearance* of multiplicity, of many forms, does not fracture the reality of Oneness.

Spiritual inquiry in this context takes for granted that the body not only has to be included in the spiritual quest, but that it is the means whereby the spiritual quest is made. From this perspective, exploring spiritual aging is exploring the embodiment of spirit, including how we can keep our bodies strong and firm enough to act as instruments of our own will in harmony with the will of the sacred consciousness.

When our quest in aging turns away from seeking a lost youth and turns towards this self, we choose the path of power and consciousness. It is a path which we walk with the body but which leads us to the spirit.

The king asked the sage,

"When the sun has set and the moon is hidden,
When the fires have all gone out and there is no sound,
What then serves as light?"

The sage answered,

"Then it is by the light of the Self
That one sits and one stands,
One comes and one goes."

THE BRHADARANYAKA UPANISHAD 4:3:6[6]

The Five Waves of Aging

It is true that scientifically we are poised on the brink of new and exciting discoveries about the human body. But the answers to the questions of aging extend beyond science to the field of our own human and personal experience. They lie within each one of us, and we must consciously bring our own experience of aging into the collective experience of humanity.

We can all take heart from Prof. Kirkwood when he says, "We have to begin to see ageing as a malleable process."[7] Its malleability will depend to a great extent on how we view it, and on how deeply we connect with the inner self – with its vitality, its resourcefulness, and its integrity. And it is to the aging body, which is the thing we have closest to hand, that we look for the secrets of the spirit. Using blood, flesh, and bone as a metaphor for the road inward, we allow the body to be the coalescence of the spirit.

Drawing from some of the great spiritual teachers of the past and from teachers of the present like Edna, I have created a map for myself that I will be sharing through this book. I have called it *the five waves of aging* because aging seems to me like taking to the sea. In youth and early adulthood we stay on a safe shore, perhaps occasionally casting a net out into the sea of the Great Unknown Spirit, but always from the safety of the well-known ground beneath our feet. Entering middle age means setting out on uncharted waters at the midday of our lives, when the sun is at its zenith and we can see both forward and backward by its light. In this light we leave behind all that we have known, while before us there is a vast horizon from which we can choose our destination. This surely is like birth, but at birth we were not making conscious choices. Now in the blazing light of the midday of our lives we can choose to begin again – *consciously*. We can choose how we navigate these waters, aware that this is the last half of this human journey, our last chance at conscious and successful living.

I call the first wave of aging "Making the Unconscious Conscious." This wave requires that as we set sail we open the storehouse of long-forgotten dreams that our body has colluded with the spirit to hide from our everyday view. We have to examine these dreams in the light of our maturity and decide how we can honor them. As we do this we develop a new relationship with bone, connective tissue, and muscle, strengthening and renewing their purpose as they reawaken to the energy of the yet to be fulfilled dream.

The second wave, "Opening Up," requires that we take up the challenge of letting go of those dreams whose time has passed. This will often mean working through resentment, bitterness, anger, and frustration – the emotions that close us down and constrict the flow of blood through our veins and arteries. Opening up to our disappointments is not giving up – it is courageously facing up to what can no longer be and moving on. The metaphor of this wave is the rhythm of the heart receiving and sending out the lifeblood of the body.

The third wave is "Staying in Touch." Living a spiritual life often requires too much isolation from other people. There is also a strong element in society that seeks to isolate the aged. In contrast to both of these, as we sail away from the shore towards a different horizon, we can stay in touch with all that it means to be human, even while we let the spirit speak and direct us. This wave demands a continued intimacy with life, even while we are letting go some of its cargo. We learn – from our remarkable sense of touch, from our nervous system hungry for stimulation – the value of being alive to life.

We also need to negotiate the fourth wave, "Re-creating Yourself." As we age and leave behind procreation, we need to re-create *ourselves*. Puberty and adolescence molded us to be the people our community or society wanted us to be – part of which meant producing the next generation of humans. Aging offers us the opportunity to be the person we ourselves want to be. We can learn from the extraordinary life of the neuron how to evolve and to be fully human.

And then we have to "Turn to Face the Other Way." Death stalks us from the moment of birth, but as we get older we feel its pace. Part of aging is facing death and the myths that we hold about it. All the previous waves will have cleared our mind to ride this wave that our heart, heeding the call of the Unlimited, is sailing towards. On the crest of this wave we look to that which is beyond the horizon, to the end of all that we know now.

As we navigate these five waves we can explore what it means to live longer on a personal level, just as science is now exploring it on a biological one. We can learn to face the challenges that aging poses by allowing the inner self to be our guide, and we can learn to make our maturity – and even our dying – a powerful and positive experience.

Beyond the Thunderdome

As I begin to offer here what I have learned, the voice of the fabulous over-60 Ms Tina Turner reminds me that the last thing we need is another hero or the way home and that we should be reaching for life beyond the Thunderdome. Aging, precisely because we are becoming successful at it, will give rise to a whole new batch of "heroes," from medical science and the pharmaceutical industry offering magic potions and pills to various experts and voices of authority and others like myself who are seeking an understanding of it.

We must remind ourselves that behind the semblance of authority there is often nothing more than fear of the unknown, and that "the way home" on offer is all too often nothing more than an impossible return to youth. Each of us must define for ourselves what aging means to us rather than reaching for someone else's "system," "method," "steps," or even "waves." Any "solution" to aging that asks us to be something other than that which we choose to be, what our spirit calls us to be, is indeed "the Thunderdome." We can reach beyond this.

There is a wonderful myth from Hinduism that might be useful to consider as we embark on this odyssey of aging. The great goddess Durga the Dreaded, she who is ever-ready to take up arms against the forces of darkness, is engaged in a terrible battle against some particularly evil opponents of truth. She slays them, but as their blood touches the earth, new and darker forces spring from it. Undaunted, the goddess allows another part of herself, Kali, to emerge from her brow, and Kali drinks the blood of the slain before it can touch the earth and give rise to new enemies.

As we age we are going to have to engage with a powerful network of media that are peddling youth. Taking a leaf from Durga's battle plan, we must learn to swallow that poison and transmute it. Take up what is useful and what you can validate through your own experience, and leave the rest behind without a backward glance, reaching for life beyond the Thunderdome.

Life has given us time and now our extended lifespan is heaping more time upon us. We can reciprocate this gift by giving purpose to this time, thereby adding aging to the list of human accomplishments. If we use our years wisely and enter into the nature and essence of aging, we will make of it something that can be looked forward to with joy.

Chapter 2

Unavoidably Present

And Krishna said,
"Know, O Arjuna, that this body is the field,
And that which knows it
Is called the Knower of the field."

THE BHAGAVAD GITA 13:1[1]

Witnessing the process of change that age brings allows us to see that there is a journey ahead for each of us. It is that witness-consciousness, which we experience as the "forever 25-year-old" within, that must now reach out and shape the journey. Rather than being drawn along life's path, it must now lead.

To begin with, we have to ensure that we have the information we need to take us beyond the shoreline of the known and out into the ocean of the unknown. The first step in that direction is to begin to participate in an expanded vision of ourselves – seeing ourselves not only as a physical body and mind on the one hand and spirit on the other, but also as a field of energy linking and engaging with both.

Energy makes everything work and fulfill the purpose for which it was created, from the stars shining across the galaxy to the electric lights in our homes and the muscles of our bodies contracting and relaxing to make breathing and movement possible. Nothing in this vast universe of ours lives or moves without energy. Every one of the trillions of cells of our body is engaged in producing energy so that we can be who we are, engage in the work we have come to do and fulfill the purpose for which we were born. And we can measure this energy by the force it exerts on matter.

However, science is now beginning to speak about another kind of energy, one that we do not have the instruments to measure. Even astronomers, a generally reserved bunch not given to making leaps of faith, have begun to theorize about an "unseen force" or "energy field" which somehow acts to sustain a "constancy" of movement in the stars and planets of the universe, a sustaining force that exists outside the measurable framework of time, space, gravity, and matter. They describe this "constancy" in terms of an invisible energy, a field of being that contains and connects us all to each other and even to the stars at the very edges of our universe. And this field is said to contain an absolutely staggering amount of energy – much more, in fact, than all the matter that exists in the universe. In other words, these scientists are admitting that the matter that we can see, that we can touch, that we can hear, is only the tip of the iceberg!

> We are poised on the brink of a revolution ... What [scientists] have discovered is nothing less than astonishing. At our most elemental, we are not a chemical reaction, but an energetic charge ... This pulsating energy field is the central engine of our being and our consciousness, the alpha and the omega of our existence.
>
> LYNNE MCTAGGART[2]

The Unseen Field

The ancient traditions of India and China have been working with this "energy," this unlimited and eternal "field," for millennia, and the names they have given it are best translated as "vitality," although they can also be translated as "life force." It is a vitality that cannot be measured and yet it can be experienced. It is independent of the cells of the body but is the essential basis of each cell, creating an organic whole in which every part communicates with every other part of every organism. And what is more, it is universal – it pervades everything, everywhere. It does not confine itself within boundaries – it is in the depths of each of us and yet it flows through the vacuum of deep space with equal force.

This vitality the Indian *rishis* (visionaries) called *prana*, a Sanskrit word which comes from a root verb that means "to fill." It fills us and it fills the space around us. Prana is not empty – it is a unifying field of vital information that is remarkably sensitive to all that we think, all that we feel, and all that we do.

The Chinese called this vitality *qi* (pronounced "chee"). The way the Chinese character for this word is structured:

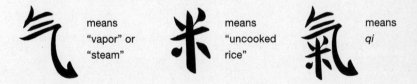

means "vapor" or "steam"   means "uncooked rice"   means *qi*

tells us something about the nature of what it refers to – it indicates the subtlety of steam, the solidity of uncooked rice, and the potential for the transformation of both the material and the ephemeral.

While to a modern scientist the body has a cellular basis, to the ancients it was this vitality, whether they called it *prana* or *qi*, that formed the basis of our being. They made a science of its study and an art of interpreting its movement, and as we age we can join these ancient visionaries and begin to look beyond the cell towards this vitality to find ourselves.

Creating a New Mind

"Never marry a man over 40," my grandmother told me one day. I was only 18 at the time and the idea of marrying a man over 40 was the farthest thing from my mind. But we grandchildren would swap Grandma's philosophies with each other with much amusement and so I asked, "Why not, Grandma?" "They're too set in their ways," she replied.

One of the things we have to work hardest at as we age is keeping our minds supple and ready to change. The easiest thing is to slip into a crusty "I've always done it this way and so I'll keep doing it this way" kind of living. Changing our minds, changing the way we see the world and ourselves, and changing the way we do things are the challenges life presents to us.

The evidence is that the view we take, the belief system we build, and the model we work to will all have a remarkably powerful impact on our aging. We have become far too committed to a common-sense view of the world – a "believe it when you see it" philosophy. However, the astonishing truth is that we organize our view of the world around our belief system, rather than reality presenting itself to our senses as it actually is.

In its constant search for stability of experience so that dangers can be recognized, our nervous system has evolved to take in only a very limited amount of information from the absolutely staggering amount all around us. Therefore our perception may be limited to a very narrow part of ourselves and the world. The scientist Sir John Eccles suggested that we actually process only about 14 per cent of all the information available to us – that means that there is a staggering 86 per cent that we are unaware of! We must begin from the point of view that we do not truly know what is out there (or in here) and, despite our age, begin again with the curiosity of a child.

> The cost of our perceived stability is over-simplification ... Our representation of reality, our beliefs and our feelings about the world, are what we act upon, not the world itself.

ROBERT ORNSTEIN AND DAVID SOBEL[3]

The Yogis of India put it another way. The mind, the senses, and the awareness, they said, collaborated to create an inaccurate picture of the universe, and our attachment to that inaccuracy represents a kind of bondage. When we are young that collaboration makes perfect sense because it allows us to take up the ambitions of our social group, to conform to them and to reproduce the human species. But as we age that collaboration begins to fall apart and something new begins to emerge, something that we experience at first as "the forever 25-year-old" within.

Expanding our awareness is what we are being called to, because then we alter both our own experience of aging and others' perception of it. Then we are truly pioneers and wizards, shamans transforming what is and creating new worlds for others to experience. In order to do this we need to accept, first of all, that we are more, much more, than can be perceived with the naked human eye. We must constantly return to the advice given to the aging disciple Uddhava and roam this world freeing ourselves from restrictive frameworks in which we think we know, in order to discover the unknown.

While science has committed itself to the study of humanity as cellular-based beings, we the aging can expand our awareness and begin to study ourselves as embodiments of the universal vitality that streams forth from the spirit. And the cell itself discloses this vitality.

Cells dividing and multiplying to evolve into tissue organizing itself into organs and systems that form our bodies are all only part of the story of life. Our cells seem to have a remarkable and finely tuned sensitivity both to our environment and to what is happening in the rest of our body at any given moment. Indeed, the life of the humble cell speaks of the unifying field of life which, far from being a mere accident of physics, has both purpose and intention.

Many writers investigating this unseen force or vitality focus on the work of a hard-working and insatiably curious character called Cleve Backster. Backster is one of America's leading lie-detector experts. He has taught the science of the polygraph machine to police academies around the country. But with his polygraph Backster has discovered a communication mechanism beyond the nerve impulses and circulatory systems that works between cells, and even between bodies that are separate from one another.

First Backster discovered that plants react when stressed and then that they react when other plants in their environment are stressed. He went on to discover that our ordinary house plants also react when we are stressed – even when we are miles away from home!

In *The Romeo Error*, a groundbreaking book that challenges the myths of dying, the scientist Lyall Watson explores the sensitivity of the cell.[4] He records an experiment in which Backster wired his electrodes to a sample of fresh human semen. Then the donor took a sniff of amyl nitrate. Amyl nitrate is a highly corrosive substance, and as it hit the man's sensitive nasal lining and began to destroy cells there, his semen – completely isolated and 40 feet away from him in a petri dish – reacted in sympathy with the dying cells in the mucous membrane of his nose.

The mystery is how these cells are communicating with one another when they are separated by space and solid walls. Their communication is clearly not confined to signals traveling along pathways of matter like nerves and synapses. If the cells of a man's semen can react from 40 feet away to the death of cells in his nasal membranes, it is not a great leap to accept the credibility of an undetectable but unifying field or vitality – the *prana* or *qi* of the ancients – that permeates every part of our being, and perhaps beyond our being, connecting us to each other and to the universe at large.

Watson also cites the work of William Tiller of Stanford University to propose a theory about how cellular communication takes place outside the nervous, hormonal, or circulatory systems of the body. Tiller uses the term "the human ensemble" to describe how humans encompass more than simply the physical body. The only way, Tiller says, that we can possibly understand cellular communication is to accept that there is more to our being than that which we can see or measure. Tiller advocates the model created by the ancient rishis of India, who postulated the existence of a number of bodies which exist alongside this measurable body of flesh and bone, and which the unseen vitality of *prana* pervades and flows through, creating an unbroken interconnectedness between them all.

This idea of this vitality is not foreign to Western cultures and was employed in medicine until the industrial revolution, when medicine itself underwent a fundamental revolution that, in embracing the new technologies, left behind much of its ancient wisdom. We lost contact with our own energy, and subtle vitality was dismissed. The great French psychiatrist Jacques Lacan points out that until Freud spoke about libido, medical theory had entirely removed energy from the human body.

The Unfolding Self

In India and China, this energy or vitality was never ignored or marginalized. The ancient Naths, a sect of Yogis that hold even the Buddha to be part of their lineage, actually created an elaborate system of chakras, or energy clusters, that they said organized this universal flow of vitality within each being. Freud organized our energy around our sexuality, but to these ancient Yogis we were made up of the stuff of the universe – space, wind, fire, earth – and it was around these that the vitality of the universe organized itself in us. This entire universe, they said, was a manifestation of an Unlimited Consciousness that expressed itself in matter through the power of *prana*.

In a timeless Indian text of just 12 simple verses called *The Mandukya Upanishad*, these ancients say that the Unlimited Consciousness manifests in three stages:

- First it unfolds to become the True Self, which is situated in the sacred space of the heart. The rhythm and cadence of this Self are closest to Unlimited Consciousness.

- It then unfolds still further to become the inner instrument, situated in the communication systems of the body. The inner instrument contains our individual consciousness, our dominant belief system, our personal identity, the way we look at the world, and therefore the way it reflects back at us.

- Finally it unfolds to become the physical body, our external instrument, that engages with creation as if it were separate from it.

Prana is the thread that runs through all three of these bodies, linking them to each other and to the Unlimited Consciousness from which they have unfolded.

The word *Upanishad* means "to sit close to." It is the teaching that was imparted to the student or seeker only after many years of study. It is a teaching that we would be mystified by in our youth, but that we are ready for as we age. We need many years of experience in order to consider the possibility that we are a constant unfolding of the infinite and that our being is the journey of the Unlimited Consciousness appearing as an individual body with awareness and personality.

However, *The Mandukya Upanishad* warns us that we must not mistake this appearance for the abandonment of our eternal and infinite nature. Just as a wave does not cease to be part of the ocean, so our individual reality does not separate us from our eternal and infinite nature. The Unlimited Consciousness, the True Self, and the body are not separate from each other.

This gives us the means of finding our way back to the Self through matter, through our physical being. In a way, this journey is the reverse of the process in which we become physical beings who go on to develop consciousness and personality. This teaching maintains that from the outset of our "coming into being" we are an entire "human ensemble" of Self, personality, identity, and body that is linked not only to this moment in time and space but also to eternity and infinity.

While Hindu in origin, this Upanishad is not contrary to other religious philosophies, and whatever our spiritual perspective, it calls on us to become more deeply involved with the life of the spirit as the source of all life.

There is in all things an inexhaustible sweetness and purity, a silence that is the fount of all action and joy. It rises up in wordless gentleness and flows out to me from the unseen roots of all created being, welcoming me tenderly, saluting me with indescribable humility. This is at once my own being, my own nature, and the gift of my Creator's Thought and Art within me ...

FATHER THOMAS MERTON[5]

The True Self

The True Self, which *The Mandukya Upanishad* calls "the Knower" (*Prajna*), is that which corresponds most closely with the Unlimited Consciousness. It is what we may more familiarly call the spirit, and it is situated in the heart. Its nature is beyond sorrow and beyond the constant to and fro of the mind. It is what we connect to and "feel" when we say we are still "25 inside."

To the ancient *rishis* this was the *bindu*, the point from which all things became possible: creation, non-creation; something, nothing, everything. As we know, once you put pen to paper, creating a point, from there you can make a straight line or a circle or a triangle or any other shape. The *bindu* is the point of emergence from which all things become possible.

Since antiquity, the *bindu* has been depicted in Indian art in complex meditational diagrams called *yantras*. These *yantras* are said to contain magical properties created to shape events to the design of their creators. They are extraordinary maps of the internal True Self, and the self which flows from it. At the center is the dot, the *bindu* that is forever the same, forever unchanging. Around it are shaped circles, triangles, polygons – all the shapes that life

takes. Look at any one of these diagrams long enough and it
appears as if one shape metamorphoses into another, changing just
as our psychological and physical world keeps changing. Only the
dot at the center remains constant.

The most elaborate of these is the *Sri Yantra*, which consists of
triangles, lines, circles, and so on, that all emanate from the center-
point, the *bindu*. This is the map the ancients left us of the cosmos
made up of individual bodies (planets, peoples, "things") and the
inner world of each individual within this cosmos.

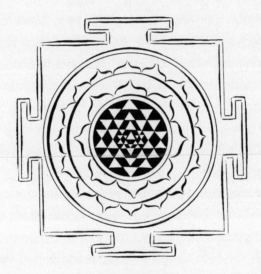

The Sri Yantra

From the point of view of meditation, it does not matter whether
you work from the outer form of the yantra and travel inwards, or
from the core and travel outwards – both journeys are valid and
both acknowledge the center as the place of emergence. Using the
five waves of aging we will be moving our consciousness from the
outer external embodiment of the self to the source point, shifting
our identification from the limited to the unlimited.

The Inner Instrument

The inner instrument is the inner light or radiance (*Taijasa*), that guides our external path. This inner light is the cognitive faculties constantly receiving information from our environment and making sense of it. It is the mind that both recognizes the information and sorts it out. It is the ego, or what the ancients called the *ahamkara* – "the idea-of-I" or "the I-maker."

In our youth and early adulthood, our awareness, what the ancients called *buddhi*, is entirely entranced by the I-maker. Its whole attention is on the external world as it makes choices to do this or that. But as we get older the I-maker begins to lose its grip and the awareness begins to expand. It begins to turn towards that True Self situated in the heart and towards that from which the True Self emerges – the Unlimited. When awareness of the True Self and of the Unlimited is complete, when the *buddhi* rests in a state of choiceless awareness, the ancients called it *buddha* – being fully awakened.

This was probably the earliest record we have of an analysis of the mind and consciousness. It is almost as ancient as upright *Homo sapiens*. As we allow our minds to reach back and be molded by this analysis, we open ourselves to an ancient part of our evolution, a time in which the spirit reached out to a fuller consciousness of itself.

The old monk whom I spoke of in the previous chapter was saying that this is where the voyage of aging may be taking us all. But awakening to our true identity is not an inevitability: we have to go consciously in that direction to get there. And we stand the best chance once we have fulfilled the demands of youth and arrived at the consciousness that comes with maturity.

The External Instrument

The external instrument is the body, *Vaishvanara*. *Vaishvanara* is not simply one's own body, it is all bodies. When we open ourselves to the idea that each individual body is an expression of the same Unlimited Consciousness as all other bodies, we approach our world in a different way. We journey towards awareness through this external instrument, this body, becoming a revelation of the True Self, the spirit, whether it is in a phase of youth or old age. That is the evolution of the spirit. We travel from the *bindu* through the maze of the internal world to the external boundary of the self.

The external instrument is part of the whole "human ensemble" – beyond muscle and bone. It is the flow of the universal *prana* or *qi*, in specific patterns and directions.

When we can see ourselves as the Unlimited, momentarily individualized but never fragmented, then we are embracing our entire human ensemble.

The Flow of Vitality

According to the visionaries, *prana* flows in a pattern that corresponds extremely closely with the physical body and even survives it after death. Running through the central axis of this pattern, where we would situate the spinal cord in physiology, is a radiant river of *prana* called *Sushumna Nadi*, the Shining Pathway. Within *Sushumna Nadi* there are a number of energy clusters called *chakras*. From these chakras flow thousands of rivers of this essential vitality that communicate with every cell of the body. And because this *prana* is universal, it informs us about everything that is happening everywhere.

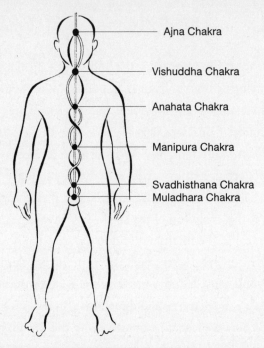

Ajna Chakra

Vishuddha Chakra

Anahata Chakra

Manipura Chakra

Svadhisthana Chakra
Muladhara Chakra

The chakras

Sushumna Nadi runs up the vertical axis of the body through the center of the spine from the perineum to the crown. On either side of it run Ida and Pingala to form a double helix resembling the structure of DNA. From each chakra nadis flow to deliver prana throughout the body.

Ajna Chakra is a powerful energy cluster that controls the chakras below it and where Ida and Pingala terminate.

Vishuddha Chakra, at the base of the neck, houses Akasha (Space) Tattva and is thus the center of organization – *prana* moving from chaos to order.

Anahata Chakra, situated behind the heart, houses Vayu (Air) Tattva and is thus the center of movement – *prana* creating both the impulse and capacity for movement in the body/mind complex.

Manipura Chakra, situated behind the navel, houses Agni (Fire) Tattva and is thus the center of transformation – *prana* empowered to change one thing into another throughout the body/mind complex.

Svadhisthana Chakra, situated at the base of the spine, houses Apas (Water) Tattva and is thus the center for creation – *prana* drawing the power of creation into each body.

Muladhara Chakra, situated at the perineum, houses Prithvi (Earth) Tattva and is thus the center of manifestation and stability – *prana* being grounded into a specific time and space.

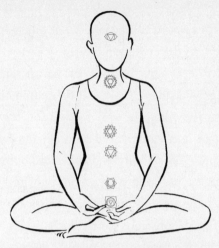

The Story of the Chakras

For thousands of years the knowledge of the chakras and thus of the pattern of the flow of *prana* through the body was held in the hands of the Nath sect, which is believed to have had its origins in Bengal and which later spread throughout India. This sect was also called the Kanpatta because of their practice of wearing heavy earrings elongating their earlobes, which eventually split. They are Hindus who worship the god Shiva as their supreme deity, but nonetheless count the Buddha as among their lineage.

Their pictorial representations of the *nadis* and chakras are usually highly stylized and were not meant to be teaching models, as the tradition of teaching they used was oral transmission from guru to disciple. It is only in the last 100 years that these teachings have begun to reach the West.

Five of the chakras, situated from the throat down to the perineum (the area where your body meets the ground when you sit), house what are called the *tattvas*. The word *tattva* literally means "that-ness" – that which makes a thing what it is, its essence. The five tattvas are:

Akasha: Space
Vayu: Air
Agni: Fire
Apas: Water
Prithvi: Earth

These tattvas are keys to our embodiment and within each of us they tell the story of the evolution of life.

Each tattva represents a force of nature and an essential process of living. Muladhara Chakra, at the perineum, holds Prithvi, or Earth, Tattva, providing the vital foundation for full emergence into the world as it is experienced through the five senses. This earthy vitality provides stability and cohesion, both psychologically and physiologically. Along with water and fire, it is the vitality that we need to engage with as we set sail on our first wave into aging: Making the Unconscious Conscious.

Water, occupying most of the planet's surface and its depths, water, from which all life emerges, is a manifestation of Apas Tattva, situated in Svadhisthana Chakra at the base of the spine. Water is the universal symbol of the unconscious, representing ancient memory as well as creativity. It holds our dreams and calls on us to bring them to the surface. Water Tattva, creating and enlivening our fluidity, holds qualities that must manifest on the first wave in our voyage into aging.

An embryo becoming a human being, or planet Earth itself transforming from a flaming ball of gas to a planet with a crust and an atmosphere able to support life, are manifestations of Agni, or Fire, Tattva, which represents transformation. Agni Tattva is situated in Manipura Chakra behind the navel and by the light of its flame we see an external world in which we appear to be separated from everything else. In our first wave we call on this tattva to point us toward a different vision by becoming aware of where we are now along our life's path.

Planets orbiting stars, stars forming galaxies, and the movement of the embryo from the Fallopian tube to the uterus are manifestations of Vayu, or Air, Tattva, which represents movement. Blood flowing freely through our arteries and veins and nerve impulses traveling at lightning speeds along our nerve pathways are all manifestations of *prana* flowing through Vayu Tattva, which is housed in Anahata Chakra, behind the heart. As we embark on the second and third waves of aging, Opening Up and Staying in Touch, we engage with the vitality of Vayu Tattva that takes us out into manifestation even while it calls on us to remain constant to the purpose of the Self within.

The fusion of sperm and egg, or the universe emerging from the chaos of the Big Bang and immediately organizing itself for life to appear are manifestations of Akasha, or Space, Tattva, which represents organization. This tattva, housed in Vishuddha Chakra at the base of the throat, is our ability to reorganize our lives around our changing bodies and changing world. As we sail the waves of Re-creating Ourselves, we connect to and use the vitality of this tattva.

Through all of these tattvas that influence the external and internal instruments, we draw close to the Knower, the point of origin in the heart, the *bindu*.

As the universal *prana* flows through us it takes on the vibration of each of the tattvas. This flow follows a different pattern in each individual. Someone who has a particularly active Akasha Tattva may be a highly organized person who has difficulty with spontaneity, while someone who has an active Agni Tattva will have great difficulty with routine and happily act on impulse. Thus while the flow of *prana* is constant through all of the tattvas, the predominance of a particular tattva distinguishes us from each other. In this way the tattvas can be seen as the notes of the symphony through which the life of matter reflects the life of the spirit.

The real achievement of this perspective is that to the ancients we were not machines separate from nature with removable and replaceable parts. We were a part of nature, and that which expresses itself through nature expresses itself through us also. We can look out at the wind picking up dry leaves and whisking them about and know that the signals traveling at breathtaking speed along our nerve pathways are a reflection of the same force, Vayu Tattva. We can gaze at the awe-inspiring mountains and mysterious valleys of Earth and know that the same force, Prithvi Tattva, exists in us as our bony structures and connective tissue. Thus we are able to see ourselves reflected in nature and let nature lead us into a deeper understanding of ourselves.

Maintaining Balance

In its ebb and flow, *prana is* subject to something the ancients called "The Law of That Which Binds." This "bondage" (*guna* in Sanskrit) applies to everything – it is the common thread, the superstring that binds together the human ensemble and all of creation, and it manifests through expansion, contraction, and equilibrium.

1. Expansion (rajas in Sanskrit) is prana in an outward movement.
2. Contraction (tamas in Sanskrit) is prana in an inward movement.
3. Equilibrium (sattva in Sanskrit) is prana at the stillpoint of balance, moving neither outward nor inward.

The best example of this law is a complete inhalation and exhalation. While we are inhaling, the body is expanding to take in air and this outward movement is *rajas*. While we are exhaling, the body is contracting and this inward movement is *tamas*. The stillpoint at the end of one exhalation and before the next inhalation is *sattva*.

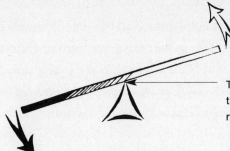

The bright *guna rajas* draws the
vitality upward and outward.

The *guna sattva* is the stillpoint,
the point of perfect balance between
rajas and tamas.

The dark, heavy *guna tamas* draws
the vitality downward and inward.

The *Gunas*: The Law of That Which Binds

The Law of That Which Binds applies to the tattvas and the chakras. For example, someone who normally has an active – *rajasic* – Svadhisthana Chakra (which houses Water Tattva) may be a deep thinker given to periods of solitude. If that same tattva then becomes *tamasic* it can express itself as depression and feelings of isolation, loneliness, and rejection. By learning to recognize these forces as we set sail into the waters of aging, we will come to a deeper knowledge of ourselves and how each of us can best express our own perfection.

In the Chinese model, this same vitality is also identified with forces of nature, however its pattern of flow is more closely associated with the major organs of the body. In both ancient India and China, longevity was a goal to be aspired to, for with it came understanding and wisdom.

Soul to Cell

If we embrace the perspective of the ancient traditions of the East, Unlimited Consciousness is seen to be embodied in us and through us. For now it is an embodied being embracing the aging process.

We can use the process of aging to draw closer to it and thus make the journey a spiritual one. This requires that we learn to connect at a deep level to the physical body, learning to see it as a vehicle that we have stewardship over while we increasingly expand our awareness of the True Self, the forever 25-year-old within.

1. As we set out on the five waves of aging, like good sailors we will learn how to prepare our boat, trim the sails, read the winds, and chart our course. With so many of us setting sail on these waters now we will surely leave traces, some whispers in the wind, that those coming after us can follow.

The First Wave

Chapter 3

Make the Unconscious Conscious

Prana, obeying universal laws, streams through the chakras in an endless flow to bring about creation – to make manifest the Unlimited. As it passes through the chakras that house Fire, Water, and Earth Tattvas it calls on us most urgently "to be" and a body that is visible and touchable emerges in space and time. Earth Tattva creates our mass, and in childhood and youth it will be in a state of dynamic ascendancy as we develop bone and muscle mass. Water Tattva will give us an ocean within, and again when we are young its flow will be strongest. Fire Tattva will give us the capacity for the transformation of growth, and in our early life is active or *rajasic*. As we age, *prana* begins to fall into a *tamasic* state in these tattvas. Its rhythm is to be in full flood in youth and to slowly withdraw and return to its source as we age.

Our lifestyle, our belief systems, and our thought processes will all influence the time and rate of withdrawal, but what will have the greatest impact is how successfully we connect to our source and how much meaning we make of our lives. *Prana* coalescing to form a solid living being does so for a purpose, and that purpose must be realized. However, just as our body forms to serve that purpose, once born, we can use it to hide the purpose – even from ourselves.

By looking at the tissue of the body that relates to Earth,

Water, and Fire Tattvas, we can begin to use the body to uncover the hidden purpose, the unfulfilled dream.

Machines cannot become like men, but men can become like machines.

ARTHUR KOESTLER[1]

The Pathways that Connect are the Ties that Bind

In our physical body, the most abundant and fundamental manifestation of the True Self is connective tissue – it is the call "to be" taken form.

At the beginning, human life is simplicity itself – three layers of cells developing from a single cell. One of these three original layers of cells is called the mesoderm and from it arises the connective tissue.

Connective tissue wraps itself around cells and penetrates them to wrap around their most minute inner parts; it is abundant in our skin and less abundant but still present in our brain. It forms unbroken plains, valleys, and mountains that provide protection and containment for cells, tissues, and organs, and connects them to each other. Connective tissue is the common element of all cells, be it of the heart, the nervous system, the eyes, or the bones. It is everywhere in the fabric of our bodies. A movement of muscle in the hand will cause a ripple in the connective tissue right up the arm and into the body. If you place your hand on your head and press down, creating pressure, you will send a signal through the connective tissue right down to the toes. Connective tissue wraps itself around an entire muscle and extends to become the tough tissue of the tendon that connects muscle to bone. The deep-course connective tissue called fascia binds muscles into functional groups and also creates a firm layer of support just beneath the skin that anchors it to underlying structures like muscle while permitting it to glide freely over them. Even our red blood cells that carry the essential oxygen to each and every cell of the body are a form of connective tissue.

Highly responsive and sensitive, connective tissue seems to be the ideal material medium for holding the purpose and dreams of a True Self as it unfolds into manifestation.

Elise's Story

Elise and I had been friends for a number of years, initially drawn together by the fact that we both had twins. She had three boys, ran a small business from home, and was happily married. Elise and her family had a comfortable lifestyle and she seemed to relish the rush and bustle of it all. Like many of my female friends, she was a true "Fire" type. Her Manipura Chakra was clearly predominant. She had careless good looks, a home that was not perfectly tidy but always bright and welcoming, and people naturally gravitated to her warmth. Her eyes had that magical light of all people with an ascendant Fire Tattva, and laughter and lively conversation always seemed to surround her.

We had arranged to meet for lunch and she was entertaining me with the tale of finally managing to get her oldest son and his beloved pet terrapins packed into the car for the trip to the university where he would be spending the next few years of his life. At first she seemed to be her usual cheerful, chirpy self, but as the lunch progressed I became aware that something was not quite right. Finally I asked, "So, what's the problem?"

She looked stricken as she said, "I'm 46 and the twins will also be going off to university next year."

I waited.

"It'll just be me and Jim and I never thought this would happen. I mean, I've never been one of those mothers who invested all of themselves in their kids, as much as I loved them, but now ..." her voice trailed off as she looked past me into the distance of an uncertain future.

This is a common story for many of us. We still by and large embrace the ambitions of our social group. This maintains a certain order in society and benefits the group as a whole – the dreams and aims of the group become our dreams also. In past generations we did not, in large numbers, live long past this period of our lives. But now, once we've been successful at achieving those parts of the group dream that we chose, we still have time on our hands. We have the house, the marriage, the family, the career, or whatever combination of these we have created, but as we enter our forties a long future still stretches ahead of us.

It took some fancy talking at lunch that day to convince Elise not to dismiss her feelings and to get her to agree to explore them fully. Women particularly are ever ready to see their own feelings and needs as somehow less valuable than those of their children, husband, or extended family. And yet it is vital that without becoming egocentric, we become ready to explore ourselves.

Elise agreed, albeit reluctantly, to spend 20 minutes twice a day going through a movement and meditation routine that I created for her. It was a routine with elements from Yoga and Chinese medicine, designed to reawaken the flow of *prana* into the chakras housing Earth, Water and Fire Tattvas and create enough space within her body for the dream to emerge. I made her promise that she would keep to the routine faithfully for three months. I also asked that during this time she watch the small, seemingly insignificant things that she did, for very often our inner voice expresses itself through tasks that we perform repeatedly but beneath the level of our consciousness.

The Unspent Dowry

Fulfilling the dreams of our social group can cause us to set aside more personal dreams. If we want to be an astronaut when we are six, our parents and relatives may point out how hard that is to achieve and then encourage us to turn our ambitions in the direction of more realizable goals. When I was six I announced at the dinner table one evening that I was going to be a priest when I grew up. Everyone burst out laughing and my father gently informed me, "Girls are not allowed to become priests." My brother always talked of becoming a writer. Instead he became a lawyer. I became a wife and a mother and worked in offices with computers to provide for my family. The dreams of childhood were stored away.

The same connective tissue that conspires with the Self to hold on to our personal dreams and help make them manifest when the time comes, simultaneously conspires with our social self, the *ahamkara*, the I-maker, to suppress and hold them down. The laughter at the dinner table when I was six sent my connective tissue into a silent wave of activity as it conspired with muscle and bone to store away the dream. Thus we use our bodies to keep our dreams alive while not yet setting them free. Then the way we stand, the way we sit, the way we gesture, all hide as much as they seek to express.

Current discussions on aging and its processes lead us to believe that either we have already fulfilled our "potential" or that it is too late. The truth is that "potential" is a mythical construction. Few of us ever reach our full potential, physical or otherwise. We might have had a greater physical potential at 20 than at 60, but what were we actually doing with that potential back then? At 20 we may have had the potential to run a marathon, but few of us did. We must now come to a full realization that it is quite possible to fulfill our potential when we are in or past middle age and even in old age. As with Edna, dreams deferred can become a reality – but first we must become aware of those dreams.

Whether you believe in genetics, Divinity, reincarnation, or a combination of these perspectives, the fact is that we do not arrive empty-handed at birth. Each of us comes into the world with certain talents, unique gifts, sometimes quite specific preferences, and *that* is our dowry. The True Self enters embodiment with these preferences and talents that are an expression of our purpose. They are the very best of what we can be – if only we have the courage.

Unfolding from a True Self which itself unfolded from the embrace of eternity, we clothe its intention with bone, muscle, and flesh which become the bearers of this dowry. And we come with more than one gift to this wedding feast called life: we are daughters and sons, mothers and fathers, partners and lovers, while simultaneously bringing energy, time, and creativity to a workplace. We can do all this because we have all the gifts necessary to be all these things. But as we reach middle age we often feel that the dowry chest is empty, that it has been spent. Our despair then communicates itself to the body, and it begins to let go of its precious cargo – connective tissue begins to break down, bones begin to waste, muscles lose bulk because they lose purpose as we lose sight of what they can still accomplish. Our despair signals the *prana* to hasten its retreat from those tattvas that provide the vitality for embodiment and we begin to lose mass – muscle mass, bone mass.

But aging can be a way to expand our choices. We may not have looked into that chest of dreams for so long that we no longer remember all that it contains. We may not have had the time as we performed the roles of family and career. But now that we are reaching middle age, assured of another 30 or 40 years or even 50, we can take up the quest again and discover our full purpose. The great privilege of aging means we are given a second chance to make our dreams come true, to live the full intention of the True Self.

So middle and old age give us the opportunity to set sail, to leave the safety of the well-known and well-worn, the dreams of our ancestors and social group, and follow the waves.

The very first wave requires that we

Make the Unconscious Conscious.

We have to reach down into ourselves and bring to consciousness the desires and dreams that have become submerged just below our level of awareness. And it is possible to do all of this without becoming negatively self-involved – though it is only possible when we have accrued the compassionate wisdom that living for a few decades in adulthood gives us.

Releasing the Arrested Dream

Being prepared to make discoveries about ourselves requires commitment. Our bodies understand commitment perfectly. We have commitment in our foundational structure: the bones that support, ground, and protect our delicate internal organs. In the first few weeks of life the body creates the blueprint for this physical foundation. From the simple connective tissue of cartilage it forms its hard resilient bones. This requires a commitment from the True Self that is conveyed to the cells and tissues of the body.

We all know that our skeleton is not one long solid bone – if it were we would not be able to move in the many extraordinary ways that we do. In fact, the skeleton is made up of about 206 bones. Any two or more bones meeting form a joint. That unseen but keenly felt *prana* streams through our joints, bridging the gaps between one bone and another, carrying information about the status of the rest of the body, about the world outside the boundary of the skin, about the feelings and thoughts flowing into and through us.

As we breathe in oxygen we breathe in *prana* from air that may have come from a rainforest continents and oceans away. *Prana* knows no boundaries. In its flow within us it finds that which is hidden deep in our joints – an old long-forgotten dream. It grasps how tissue all around the joint has colluded to keep the dream alive but shut out, because at some time in our past we were unable to bring that part of ourselves to full expression. Taking its direction from body tissue, this *prana* begins to divert itself around the joint rather than flowing through it. Thus the joint becomes starved of its most basic cosmic nourishment, just as it is starved of the vital nutrients it needs from the blood.

We need to create the space within ourselves for our forgotten dreams to emerge. The ancient Yogis observed that the body contracts, making small and closing off those spaces that usually allow vitality to flow freely. They called this the distressed state – *dukha*. *Dukha* is emotional and psychological, and it is manifest in the outer instrument as the tightening and hardening of the tissues around joints and in muscles that inhibits movement.

The ancients offered us a different way of organizing the body, a way free from distress, in which we create and expand into space, and they called this expressive state *sukha*. Modern body-workers, the heirs of the ancient Yogis, work very much on the same principle. They enable the body to create space around tissue that has become compressed by tension and trauma. Ironically, the German word *Traum* means "dream!"

In the presence of the downward pull of gravity which our muscles resist, we also organize our bodies around the experiences we encounter in living a life. While gravity, responding to the imperative of Earth Tattva, pulls us down, our muscles, responding to the call of water, fire, wind, and space, are pulling us up so that we can move along the Earth's surface. The muscles that have taken on tone to keep us up respond in this state of alertness to the other forces in our environment. When we pull back a dream, for example because our parents warn that it is impossible, connective tissue, bone, and muscle conspire to hold it for us. We cannot express it, but we have not consciously let it go – and the body takes this into account every time it moves. The tension in connective tissue and muscles exerting a force on bone is what our intention to move – whether to open a door or pick up a child – encounters. We may not be aware of it, but that tension remains until we become conscious of the suppressed dream and release it.

As gravity pulls down and skeletal muscles pull up, a counter-poise is created that can be perfectly balanced and beautiful to look at: *rajas* and *tamas* in perfect balance. A body in this posture is a body of vitality in which movement continues to remain a possibility.

However, bone responds to the pull of these two forces by laying down more bone where the stress is greatest. Thus repeated movement can cause bone mass in certain areas to become dense even while we are losing mass in others – just as remaining in one set of responses to life's changes can cause our personality to harden and lose adaptability. Bone, taking its cue from connective tissue and muscle, organizes itself to support and protect our dreams, allowing them the solidity of rock to anchor themselves to – or, if they are ignored long enough, to become petrified!

Our resistance to change is really a resistance to changing ourselves and our responses to the world. For example, when we resist our children growing up and leaving home it is often because we are resisting the idea of becoming something other than a mother or father – we are resisting the opportunity for personal evolution and change that life is offering.

A Conscious Act of Will

It was the evolution of the skeletal muscle structure that allowed us to stand up and survey the distant horizon. From the moment we did that as a species we were on the move – out of Africa and into the rest of the world. Muscle, more than any other "organ" of the body, can be said to represent our will. After all, it is muscle that will take us out for a walk, or let us boogie the night away, or let us just curl up for an evening with a good book.

Smooth muscles (also called involuntary muscles) line the walls of our blood vessels and internal organs and carry out their functioning without our conscious input. The heart is a powerful smooth muscle that acts of its own volition. But muscle attached to the bones of our skeleton is under our conscious control. Yet, astonishingly, 90 per cent of the activity of this skeletal muscle is happening subconsciously in response to our intent.

For example, usually when I reach to open a door I do not consciously choose which arm will go forward to grasp the handle. I don't have to relay instructions to every muscle or group of muscles involved about when to contract and when to release. I don't have to consciously calculate the kind of force needed to turn the handle. Underneath the surface of my awareness my body makes all these calculations for me in response to my intention to open the door. A wave of activity flows through connective tissue, muscle, and bone in response to my intention.

What then, when that intention is to house a dream, a wish, a means of total self-fulfillment? Vitality that could enable our muscles to implement the conscious direction of the nervous system is being tied up by the unconscious direction to keep our dreams bound. This is not an environment of fluidity and flexibility – it is the barren environment of rigidity. Gradually the tattvas of Earth, Fire, and Water will decline into tamasic states and this barren rigidity will manifest as tightened, fibrosed muscle, an exhausted nervous system and loss of bone and muscle mass.

Restoring Balance

Elise had been doing her routine for about two months when we discussed her progress. She said it felt good to be sticking to a routine, but she could not understand how it would help her become aware of a self that was below a conscious level. During our discussion she mentioned someone she had never spoken of before – her grandmother. I knew Elise's father had died when she was young but what she volunteered that day was that since her mother had to work while she was growing up, she used to go to her grandmother's three days a week after school – and this was not a pleasant experience. Apparently Bessie, the mother of her mother, often reminded Elise what a burden the death of her father had placed on her mother. I asked Elise to invite her grandmother, who had passed away 20 years earlier, into her walking exercise (covered in the next chapter).

About a month later when Elise phoned me she was very animated and talking very quickly. She had noticed that when she was talking on the phone she would doodle, as many of us do. But while most people's doodles are a jumble of shapes, Elise's would be an eye or a nose or a mouth that was easily recognizable as that of a friend or of one of her sons or her husband. Now she said, "I wanted to be an artist."

Elise's father had been an artist who had used his self-taught skills to earn a living as a sign painter. But it seems that every time Elise had taken out her pencils and crayons to draw, her grandmother would scold her and send her back to her schoolwork.

Elise and I got together and discussed her recollections of herself and her grandmother. As she talked about that time it gradually dawned on Elise that in every other way her grandmother had been a loving and kind person. But the position the old lady had adopted in response to Elise's desire to express herself artistically had evoked such a powerful resistance in her body that it had clouded her memory of her. Elise wept copiously that day as the tension flooded from her body and she held in her consciousness the buried treasure – a dream to reproduce the world in lines and color on paper.

Back to the Garden

When we are making the unconscious conscious, we must ask ourselves the question God asked of Adam and Eve in the Garden of

Eden after they had eaten the fruit from the Tree of Knowledge: "Where are you?" We have to assume God asked not because He did not know, but because it was a question they had to consider.

We too have to consider the fundamental question: Where am I? Where am I in relation to where I started out? I came with a full dowry of gifts to this life – where am I along *that* path?

Like Adam and Eve, the answer all too often is that we are hiding. We are seeking not to face what and who we are – and therefore we cannot face the True Self.

Nevertheless the True Self will appear in one form or another and ensure that that question is asked. For Elise it was her children leaving home and the prospect of an empty house and unfilled hours. For someone else it might be the ending of a career or the thought of retirement just over the horizon, while for another it may be a marriage or long-term partnership suddenly dissolving. Each age, each time, will bring the question in its own form – and each time we will have to expose ourselves, face expulsion from Eden, the garden of our comfort zone, and work our way back to a truer Eden, one that we are co-creators of. We have the means to do so. Like Adam and Eve our nakedness may be exposed, but through that body our dream may also be revealed.

As we move on to look at what it means to ride this first wave of aging, we will look at the kind of activities we need to engage in to open up our unconscious dreams and reinforce the flow of *prana* through the tattvas of Fire, Water, and Earth to bring vitality to our renewal of purpose.

Chapter 4

Riding the Wave of Making the Unconscious Conscious

Once we have understood that concealed within and guarded by the body are a host of dreams that house our purpose for being, we have to assume the responsibility of bringing those dreams to consciousness. This means handling our lives and our activities in a wholly different way – making time and bringing a creative awareness to the sensations of the body that is waiting to reveal the purpose of the spirit. Like Edna and Elise, if we are serious about aging with spirit we have to embrace practices that move us closer to the heart of our being.

To ride this first wave we need to honor both the internal and the external instruments. That means honoring the spirit of connective tissue, bone, muscle, and our internal ocean. We also have to ensure that our mental and emotional capacities of creativity, inner vision, and transformation are balanced. Connective tissue, bone, and muscle are created to move – to hold and to release. The chakras associated with them will be activated by the physical, mental, and emotional movements we make. If we fail to call upon the flow of *prana* through these centers by leading a sedentary lifestyle or letting our mental and emotional responses become stuck, these chakras will draw less and less *prana* from the universal flow and we will lose body mass, ease of movement, and spiritual poise.

Engaging in conscious movement means that a world of personal dreams and deeply held purpose that we suppressed as we were growing up will once again reveal itself to us.

The first responsibility is to restore movement to our bodies and minds and bring sensitivity and time to that movement. That is what riding this first wave means.

Movement and Bone

Ceasing to move, lethargy of body and mind, is an indication that we no longer connect to the vitality of our dreams. As long as we are acting on the impulse of dreams which the Self became embodied to unfold, we move with the full force and strength of spiritual purpose impelling us. Disconnecting from that purpose brings about tiredness and lethargy.

Throughout our lives our bones keep remodeling themselves. Hormones produced in the parathyroid and thyroid glands stimulate the body either to break down bone and release calcium into the bloodstream or to store calcium in the bones and thus build them up. A process called "Wolfe's Law" means that bone grows in response to the forces or demands placed on it. In other words, the consequence of being sedentary is that the bones are not being stressed by movement and activity and will therefore not require any build-up. On the other hand, movement and coping with the downward pull of gravity place the bones under stress so that they have to build up.

As we age, our bones lose mass. If this loss becomes too great we are in danger of suffering from osteoporosis, a condition in which our bones become porous and vulnerable to breaking. The speed of the loss of bone mass is determined by several factors, and movement is one of the major ones. A research program at the University of Wisconsin determined that even 80-year-olds confined to wheelchairs were able to increase both bone and muscle mass with simple arm and leg exercises. Diet is another important factor in determining bone mass. Smoking, heavy drinking, excess salt, caffeine, and sugar all promote bone loss, and part of our spiritual journey as we age must be to re-evaluate our diet and become informed about what our body needs in order to continue to grow.

The point at which movement takes place is the joint, where one bone meets another. A particularly tough but highly flexible type of connective tissue called cartilage protects most joints. Made up of 80 per cent water, cartilage is able to cushion our joints when we are standing, walking, or running, shaping itself to suit our activities.

Aging can often cause inflammatory conditions of the joints known as arthritis. Osteoarthritis is the "wear and tear" arthritis that is quite common in middle and old age. It refers to the breakdown and roughening of the cartilage at the joints. As this breakdown continues, the exposed bone thickens and forms bony spurs that enlarge the bone ends and restrict movement. Rheumatoid arthritis is an inflammatory condition of the joints that can begin at any age. It starts off as an inflammation of the membrane of the joint that then thickens and begins to adhere to the cartilage, causing it to erode and form scar tissue. In both of these conditions, and as a preventive for them, we have to remember the importance of movement. Cartilage is avascular – it has no direct blood supply of its own – and it receives nutrients only when joints undergo their full range of movement.

Movement and Muscle

By adulthood, water makes up half of our mass. Muscle makes up most of the other half. There are basically three types of muscle tissue in the body: skeletal, cardiac, and smooth. Skeletal muscle is the most widely distributed muscle – it powers our movement and acts at the command of our will. This form of muscle also maintains our posture, stabilizes our joints, and gives heat to our body through the energy produced when it contracts – that is why we become warm when we exercise.

Just as bone mass tends to decrease as we age, so does muscle mass. However, using muscle continuously increases its mass and strength. We know that this increase can continue as long as we are alive and as long as we keep moving right and eating right.

Connective Tissue and Movement

Our entire being is interlaced by connective tissue at every level of our physical existence, creating a fantastic network that supports, binds, and connects. Some kinds of connective tissue, like cartilage, have no direct blood supply of their own, while other types have only a meager blood supply and yet others a very rich one. Movement and muscular activity give connective tissue the warmth and energy it needs to maintain fluidity. When any part of the body loses mobility, the connective tissue in the area loses its fluidity, resilience, warmth, and life.

Connective tissue draws *prana* from all three of the chakras we have been working with in this section: Earth provides its mass, Water its fluidity, and Fire its remarkable ability to be so many things to the single body.

The Internal Ocean and Movement

Water floods our cells and the minute spaces between our cells. Watery plasma flowing through our veins and arteries carries red and white blood cells for distribution throughout the body. Cerebrospinal fluid held within the cranium and part of the spine bathes the space around the brain with an endless tide of water that has its own sacred rhythm.

For us to remain properly hydrated, our water intake must equal our output. In a normal adult under normal conditions that is about 2,500 ml in a 24-hour period. Most water enters our body through what we drink and eat. We lose water through urine, feces, perspiration, and even breathing out. On hot days or days when we perspire through exercise we need to increase our water intake to make up for the loss.

As blood flows through the body, watery plasma leaks from the tiny capillaries into the space surrounding the cells. The body then needs to gather up this fluid and deliver it back into the circulatory system as speedily as it can. The mechanism for doing this is the lymphatic system, which, unlike the circulatory system, has no pump driving it. Lymph fluid therefore relies entirely on movement, even the movement of breath, to push it back towards the heart.

Drawing on *Prana* through Movement

In order to give bone, connective tissue, muscle, and the internal ocean the best chance of retaining their properties of life, you must engage in movement, especially weight-bearing movement.

Because your body itself has weight, brisk walking is an excellent form of movement to encourage the laying down of mass in the bones and muscles. As we age, our joints, particularly our knee joints, lose some of their cushioning effect, and therefore walking can very often be better exercise than running or jogging. Ensure that you adopt a fairly brisk pace, moving at about three miles an hour and keeping your arms swinging. This means you will be breathing more heavily than usual but would probably still be able to carry on a conversation. Walking in this way on a daily basis for 20 minutes will also tone up and strengthen the muscles of the abdomen, legs, and buttocks, and restore fluidity to connective tissue.

Movement and the Balance of Vitality

Movement draws *prana* into Manipura Chakra that houses Fire Tattva (as the muscles warm up from the movement), into Svadhisthana Chakra that houses Water Tattva (as the body becomes rehydrated through movement), and into Muladhara Chakra that houses Earth Tattva (as bone is called upon to strengthen and renew itself).

Muladhara Chakra also governs our sense of balance – one of the major "markers" of biological aging. When you try and balance, the body calls *prana* from its universal source into itself, right down to Earth Tattva at the perineum, so add to your routine this sequence of balancing postures to enhance the flow of vitality (see opposite).

To begin to draw close to the dreams that your body has held for you in safekeeping you can do a walking meditation that further contributes to the free flow of prana and will draw you closer to experiencing your entire "human ensemble."

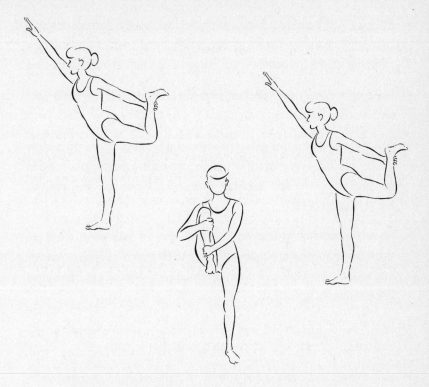

Balancing movements: Nataraj to Crane and back to Nataraj

Touching the Dream and the Walking Meditation

All of your experiences from the moment of conception have been filtered through the *ahamkara*, the I-maker, and it has created an identity out of those experiences. The *buddhi*, self-awareness, has been entranced by this I-maker (even though it may be beginning to suspect there is something more to life). Now we are going to give the *buddhi* its first conscious exercise in stepping back from the I-maker to observe its construction.

• Once you have done your brisk 20-minute walk, slow down the pace and continue to walk but in a slow, self-aware manner. Self-observation is now the primary task.

- Be aware of your breathing slowing down, your heartbeat slowing down, your muscles releasing. Begin to feel the contact your feet are making with the ground as you slowly put one foot in front of another.

- Become aware of your contact with the air by feeling it against your skin and as you breathe.

- Ask yourself if you feel safe where you are walking. If you do, simply continue; if not, ask yourself where you would feel safer and resolve to go there tomorrow and resume this exercise. Once you feel safe you are able to proceed.

- Allow yourself to go backward in time and let your mind alight on someone from your childhood. It's best to let the mind choose quickly and take the very first person it comes up with, without engaging in an internal debate about it.

- Now feel that this person is walking beside you. Let yourself go deeply into the image of this person being beside you.

- With this person walking beside you, become intensely aware of yourself and how your body/mind posture has changed. How do you feel walking with this person beside you – is it pleasant or unpleasant?

- Allow all the feelings associated with this person to flow through your consciousness and be keenly aware of the physical sensations that these feelings evoke as you walk.

- As you become aware of these physical sensations, ask yourself where in your body you are carrying the memory of this person. Fragments of memory might be stored in many places. Give yourself time to allow them to emerge. (For example, when Elise did this walking meditation her grandmother was the first person to spring to mind and she felt her body become uncomfortable and tense, particularly her jaw, shoulders, and arms.) If the person is a pleasant and loving companion who evokes feelings of tenderness or love rather than tension, enjoy these feelings and still remain aware of where and how your body has stored them.

- Without discontinuing your walk, begin to breathe into the places where you feel any particular tension. This is your past. You are not discarding it, you are honoring it. The way in which you organized your experiences of this person is the way in which your inner instrument, *Taijasa*, the Radiant Being, colluded with your body to protect you. Honor that by letting the memory remain there, whether pleasant or unpleasant, but continue to breathe into the tense area, allowing it to soften and come to rest. It might take a few walks to accomplish this, but remember that time is now on your side.

- It may happen that you go into fight-or-flight mode. If so, discontinue the session and head home rather than evoke a powerful and negative response. But make a commitment to return to this memory and this person to explore where they are in you when you feel stronger.

- After a few "walks" with this person, let yourself gradually begin to process your experience of them. You now know your responses to them. Processing these feelings allows you to understand how they made you, how they formed your idea-of-I.

- Avoid becoming analytical in this processing. Remain a passive observer of all of your responses to the memories that surface, and continue to breathe into the areas where you experience physical sensation.

Throughout your meditation remember you are learning about the *ahamkara* – the idea of I – that was shaped by the people and influences that surrounded you as you were growing up and coming into being. The ahamkara is meant to be a reflection of the True Self but often the reflection becomes clouded by those influences and it forgets its true nature. The walking meditation is one of the methods for beginning to clear that mirror.

The great Eastern sage Patanjali said that observation in itself brings about change. It takes great courage to stay with this kind of observation because sometimes the memories evoked are frightening and traumatizing. When you feel too overwhelmed to carry on, remind yourself of your maturity, of all the years that you have lived and survived in spite of this memory – maybe in some strange way even because of it. Remind yourself of all you have done and all that you have accomplished and overcome in your years. Give yourself loving time to take these walks with the past.

• When you are able to walk with the person and feel no physical reaction to their presence then you have probably processed all that you can of them for now. On your next walk let your mind choose another person.

In this way work through a list of people who have had a great influence on you, for better or worse. You will be evoking memories of those who either encouraged or caused you to set aside those unconscious dreams. By entering once more into your relationship with them, you will be re-engaging with your earliest self – that part of you which cherished those dreams and the true purpose which you came with.

In addition to movement, bone, connective tissue, and muscle need to be given time and focused attention on a daily basis in order to release tension. Wilhelm Reich, one of the most respected body-workers of the 20th century, claimed that when muscle became over-burdened by tension it would begin to release that tension inward into organs and this was a catalyst for organ diseases like cancer. At the very least, failure to release tension from muscles means that the flow of vitality is caught up in maintaining that tension rather than being available to you. The following exercise will help you to release tension.

Tension Release

As this exercise contains a number of instructions, you might like to record it on tape and then listen to it as you do the exercise.

I recommend starting from the Alexander Supine Position, as it places the body in the very best possible position to facilitate a release of tension.

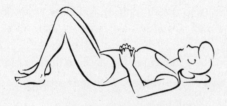

Alexander Supine Position

- Once you are in the Alexander position you will be looking up at the ceiling. Keep your eyes open for a moment and then slowly close them, feeling the lids meeting.

- Let your eyelids rest for a second or two, then slowly open them again and slowly close them again.

- Repeat this a few times, taking your time and feeling the difference in the amount of effort it takes to open your eyes and the amount of effort it takes to close them. Then let your eyes close and rest.

- Turn your attention to the contact you are making with the support beneath you – at the back of your head, your shoulder blades, your elbows – and then take your awareness down through your back, feeling the places where it makes contact with the ground, especially at the back of your hips and buttocks. Feel the contact the soles of your feet are making with the ground.

- As you breathe out, feel that you are releasing your whole weight through these points of contact into the ground.

- Feel your weight flowing through these points of contact, through the mat or carpet you are lying on, through the floor and through the structure of the building into the rich, dark earth.

- Feel the earth welcome your weight and offer its support willingly as with each exhalation you release more and more weight into the ground beneath you.

- Become aware of any tension in your scalp, around your temples and in your forehead, and slowly and consciously allow that tension to ease away.

- Become aware of any tension in the delicate tissue around your eyes, and as you let that ease away, sense that a feeling of deep peace and calm is flowing into your ears.

- Become aware of your jaw. If your teeth are clenched together, let them slowly part and let your jaw relax but keep your lips together so that you keep breathing through your nose.

- Become aware of any feelings of tension or tightness in your throat and breathe in deeply, feeling that your breath is like the wind picking up dry leaves in fall. Breathe out, letting the out-breath take the tension with it. Repeat this until the throat feels relieved of tension.

- Allow the muscles in the back of your neck to soften and lengthen, and let the muscles of your shoulders release and widen.

- As your shoulders continue to release, feel your entire chest expanding and opening, and your arms sinking down and releasing into their support.

- Be aware of the contact your hands are making with your abdomen and let your palms and fingers release, open and lengthen.

- Take your attention again to your abdomen and your back. Breathe in deeply and allow any tension from these areas to release as you breathe out.

- Feel your awareness sink down into your pelvis and let the breath follow your attention. Allow the pelvis to open as you breathe in, and as you breathe out feel the tension flowing from it and let this feeling of release travel round to the back of your hips and buttocks.

- Feel your hips and buttocks sinking down deeper into the support beneath them as they release the tension.

- Take this feeling of release down to your thighs, through your knees, down through your lower legs and ankles right down into your heels and along your feet into your toes.

- As you feel your feet sinking deeper into the support beneath them, feel that your knees are floating up towards the ceiling.

- Take your awareness back to your hands resting on your abdomen and feel that the backs of your hands have grown light and soft, rising like puff pastry.

- Take your awareness back to the crown of your head and feel that as your feet release down, the crown of your head is flowing upward.

- Let yourself stay in this place of quiet release for a couple of moments as you observe your breathing – not trying to breathe in any special way, simply becoming the observer of the sensations of breathing and resting.

- Let this observation become particularly focused on the moment between the exhalation and the next inhalation – the stillpoint.

- Become aware of that stillpoint and watch keenly for the very first movement that gives rise to the next breath.

This whole exercise of release should take no more than 10 minutes. Once you have completed it, bend your knees and roll over. You might like to take a minute to add to your routine the following breathing technique that will enliven Earth, Water, and Fire Tattvas, or you may

prefer to sit up slowly. Give yourself a moment or two to experience
the sensations of your body fully before you go back into the activities
of the day.

The Enlivening Breath

- Remain aware of your breath, feeling the sensations of cool air entering your nose as you breathe in and warm air rising up through your
  throat as you breathe out.

- Let your awareness flow down to the base of your spine, rooted deep
  in your pelvic basin; then feel it flow up your back, between your
  shoulder blades, up the back of your neck, right up into your skull and
  up to the crown of your head.

- Once you have connected to your spine, take your awareness down to
  your perineum and fix your attention there.

- As you breathe in, feel that the in-breath is entering through the space
  between your legs, contacting first the Earth Chakra at the perineum.
  Feel the cool in-breath flowing into the end of the spine at the tailbone
  to contact the Water Chakra, and like a river continuing through the
  base of the spine to the Fire Chakra in the spine behind the navel.

- As you breathe out, feel the warm air flowing back down from the Fire
  Chakra, through the Water Chakra, and out through the Earth Chakra.

- Begin to allow your pelvis to move gently with the breath just as your
  chest moves with the breath. As you breathe in, let your hips tilt gently
  back onto the floor and your tailbone lift, and then let them release as
  you breathe out. Let yourself become aware of all the sensations of
  this movement.

- With each breath feel that the chakras are becoming energized and
  that their vitality is flowing freely up and down your spine and from
  there through your body with each breath.

We all have to engage in everyday tasks like washing dishes, cleaning drawers, and walking the dog that do not require a great deal of thought. Often, while part of us is engaged in these tasks, the mind slips into a state that is natural to it. Observing the unguarded moment can offer insight into our hidden dreams and purpose.

Observing the Unguarded Moment

Try to find out where your mind goes, what it alights on in those unguarded moments.

Or, when something new happens to you, what does your mind do with the information – how does it process it?

Record your observations in a notebook – you will be amazed at what you will uncover about yourself.

Once you have begun these movement programs and exercises, Earth, Water, and Fire Tattvas will have awakened from a tamasic state and become ready for deeper meditative work.

Connecting with the Dream: Where Am I?

This is a 20-minute meditation. Ensure that the telephone is off the hook and that family members, if they are around, know that you do not want to be interrupted for this time.

- Find a comfortable chair that allows your back, neck, and head to flow in a straight line rather than a slouch.

- Close your eyes and become aware of your weight flowing down through your sitting bones into the chair and through the chair into the ground beneath you.

- Feel your weight also flowing down through your legs into the floor.

- Let your shoulders release and widen, and become aware of the muscles at the back of your neck softening and lengthening and your jaw relaxing.

- Begin to feel your contact with the air through the breath. Feel the cool air enter your nose, hit the back of your throat and warm as it enters your lungs. Feel the warm air rising up your throat and leaving through your nose.

- Follow the out-breath to the pause between breaths. Maintain awareness in that pause, watching for the very first movement that gives rise to the next breath.

- Let your mind go back, back, back along that road to its beginning, its *bindu.* From that point at which your life began you stepped onto a certain path.

- Once you have established that pathway behind you, ask yourself quite simply, "Where am I now in relation to where I started out?"

- Simply observe the images that the mind presents to the awareness.

You are simply inquiring of your inner wisdom, of the Inner Self, if where you are now is where you are meant to be.

If you are, great, open your eyes and celebrate.

If you feel that you have got sidetracked along the way and, however enjoyable those sidetracks were, you have not arrived at the point where your original purpose wanted you to be, you need to investigate further.

Important Points to Remember in this Meditation

- The *ahamkara*, which is what would have allowed itself to become sidetracked, will seek to defend itself in all kinds of ways. The most destructive is the way it acts as the policeman within. To overcome this, do not seek to understand or justify your present situation, simply become aware of it.

- Identify your feelings about where you are now.

- Accept that these feelings are real and valid without judging them as good or bad.

- Begin to experience these feelings as energy that has either propelled you forward or held you back.

- Make a journal about the experience once your meditation is complete.

Through these exercises you are awakening the powerful three chakras of being in the world. You have begun your journey at the outermost part of yourself, the most visible expression of who you are: flesh and bone. By approaching these as a continuum of the spirit, the Self within, you have entered into a new relationship with your body and drawn *prana* back into the energy clusters that serve it.

You are also learning to create some distance between your awareness (*buddhi*) and the I-maker (the *ahamkara*), thus training yourself in conscious awareness. Once you have committed to uncovering where you are, you are ready to move on to the next wave, that of Opening Up.

The Second Wave

Chapter 5

Open Up

The Light of the Unlimited shines above all things in heaven
and on earth.
It is beyond us and yet it is at the center of the heart.
It is the warmth of our body
And the sound that is heard when the ears are closed.

THE CHANDOGYA UPANISHAD 8:1:2[1]

The heart, leaning in from the left, sits in the center of the chest. Embraced by the soft tissue of the lungs and protected by the hard bone of the spine at the back, the breastbone in the front, and the ribs all round, it connects and integrates the entire body via arteries, veins, and capillaries. Thus to the Chinese physician the heart is the "emperor organ" and to the Yogi it is the center of the True Self. Vayu Tattva, the tattva of Air, is housed in Anahata Chakra behind the heart and creates the impulse for movement that allows the point, the *bindu,* to move outward towards creation. One of its impulses in the physical body is the beating heart.

The heart sends oxygen and nutrients to every cell, feeding tissues and collecting waste through its persistent and regular rhythm. Its sacred beat gives our minds the nourishment to think and our muscles the ability to move. We feel the inner cadence of the heart change when we reach out in compassion or retract with rejection.

No bigger than our fist, the pear-shaped heart rules the ebb and flow of vitality just as it rules the ebb and flow of blood. As an emperor it is a humble and obliging sovereign; as the center of the True Self it is the knowing awareness. When it stops beating, all the organs of the body, deprived of oxygen and nutrition, slowly grind to a halt. Heart and circulatory diseases are the primary killers in the Western world. The heart, it seems, demands from us a life well lived.

When there is a failure of the arteries, capillaries, and veins, the conduits that deliver the living connective tissue that we call "blood," the heart is threatened. It relies on these rivers for its own functioning as much as any other cell or tissue in the body. What are the processes that close these arteries down? What message does an open, receptive artery signal, and what is its prayer as its outer walls harden and its inner walls become furred and clogged? What halts the impulse of Vayu Tattva?

As we grow older we use connective tissue, muscle, and bone to defend the heart. Our shoulders rotate forward, our chin pushes out to lead the head forward, and slowly we close ourselves in around a heart that is closing down. Having unfolded from a single point in infinity to become human beings, we begin to withdraw, retreating from pain, disappointment, and loss, to fold ourselves around the receptacle of our pain rather than our infinite origin. We close ranks against too many blows, too many shattered dreams, too many defeats, too many broken promises given and received. We cease to expect the best and keep only the most pitiable embers of our youthful hopes burning deeper and deeper within the chambers of our heart, hidden from a world that we feel is waiting to wound us again.

The Ancient Heart

Many thousands of years ago, Chinese, Egyptian, and Indian physicians felt the heart's rhythm in the pulse in order to read the general state of health or disease of the whole body. Elaborate ceremonies would surround this reading, which was always considered a sacred act. Sometimes the physician would spend hours with his fingers resting lightly on his patient's wrist (the radial pulse) as he waited for the heart to yield up the secrets of the body. If we in our modern, technologically sophisticated world want a deeper understanding of the heart that is failing us, perhaps we need to turn to these ancient healers for guidance.

The pulse, the rhythm of the heart, would indicate to the ancient physician the quality of the vitality as it flows through the organs and the mental and emotional state of the person. For example, when I took the pulse of a friend who had bowed her body and mind around an incident in her past that she considered a betrayal, it was slow and sinking. This told me there was a heart Yang deficiency alongside an obstruction to the flow of vitality. In Western medicine this may translate as atherosclerosis – fatty deposits lining the arteries that take the blood from the heart to the body. It also indicated that psychologically my friend had lost the will to act – the impulse that propelled her forward on her life-path had become smothered.

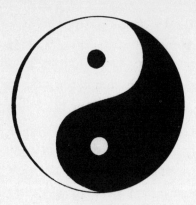

The Yin/Yang symbol

As the blood courses through the veins and arteries to and from the heart, it needs to move freely and smoothly. When it does so, a physician placing a stethoscope on the heart can hear the reassuring and repetitive lubb-dub beat of the heart's valves opening and closing. But when the arteries become clogged the heart must work harder, pushing with greater force in order to keep supplying that life-giving liquid to the body in need of it. Our blood pressure then rises and under that pressure the heart itself becomes labored, its rhythms and sounds change, even its size can change. It works hard not to fail us, but all too often we fail it.

Joe of the Mighty Heart

I first met Joe when he came to consult me about whether acupuncture would help ease the tinnitus he had been suffering from for some years. Tinnitus is a maddening ailment that impairs the hearing as the sufferer has a constant noise sounding in the ears all the time – anything ranging from a drone to a high-pitched whistle. Joe had been suffering from it for four years.

Joe's childhood dream, it emerged in the sessions that followed, had been to fly, and that is what he had accomplished. For 12 years he had lived his dream as a pilot for a large airline and then, after insulin-dependent diabetes had set in, he was professionally grounded. He still flew, however, obtaining a private license and spending weekends in the air away from his desk job.

On further examination I learned that Joe also suffered from hypertension, high blood pressure. He was grappling with two of the most sinister "silent" killers of our time. It is estimated that vast numbers of mature adults are walking around with undiagnosed diabetes and/or hypertension and are thus at risk of a sudden stroke, heart attack, or coma. Joe's hypertension was almost certainly a response to the diabetes, which often creates long-term vascular problems like atherosclerosis due to raised levels of blood cholesterol.

Seven months after Joe's regular pilot's physical had uncovered the diabetes, his wife had left him for someone else. They had been childhood sweethearts; she was his only love and the thought that they would one day part had never entered Joe's mind. But while he had been flying around the world, his wife had been left to bring up their daughter on her own, and, as Joe saw it, this had made her lonely and vulnerable to any predatory male around.

Joe's posture was always rigid, his jaw and fists often clenched tight. Such a posture would not have come simply from the past few years but would have taken a lifetime to achieve. When he talked about the break-up of his marriage he would articulate through clenched teeth. Joe was angry and he had been angry for a long time.

Joe had organized himself around an anger that he physically kept under tight rein. Muscles worked and strained to keep it in check. With this posture Joe was defending his heart and in the process putting it at risk.

After some time, as we discussed his marriage, Joe slowly came to the realization that quite possibly it was not only his frequent absences while working that made his wife lonely, but also the fact that he was unable to make himself emotionally available to her. Joe, who would risk flying a flimsy single-seater plane to dizzying heights, was afraid of admitting to his wife just how much he loved her and how dependent he was on her love and support. It is not that Joe did not love – he loved mightily and the sheer power of it frightened him because it made him vulnerable. Thus, probably at a young age, he had so disconnected from all the feelings associated with his heart that he was now closing it down. Rather than spending time on what in his past had caused this, we focused on what in the present could change it. Joe began doing many of the exercises you will find in the next chapter.

Like the ancient Eastern physician for whom the beat of the heart taps out the ailments of the body, we need to be able to listen to our heart and let it yield up the secrets of our lives. This brings us to the second wave, that calls on us to

Open Up.

The heart is in perpetual motion, taking oxygen-rich blood from the lungs to distant cells via the arteries and receiving from the veins the blood that has released its oxygen to the body. In this way the body communicates with the heart and the heart with the body. But when we cease to be open to life's changes – in ourselves, our families, our friends, our communities, the world – we begin to interrupt the smooth flow of life and this blockage is expressed in the diminished flow of blood through our arteries and veins. We begin to adopt a lifestyle that supports this shut-down: a high-fat diet, smoking (the slow suicide), high stress, too much alcohol, etc.

In truth, we can hide nothing from ourselves and, through the flow of the universal vitality, life hides nothing from us. Life will continue to touch us, however much we try to close off to the touches that are bruising. If we stay open, pain can become the path-maker of joy, and we can begin to live as we grow up and grow old.

To the physicians of India and China, whose sight relied as much on the inner vision powered by Fire Tattva as it did on photoreceptors of the eye, the heart is the vessel through which we become manifest. As they saw it, primordial, unmanifest, unlimited consciousness exists in a profound and blissful silence, which they called anhad. Anhad is the wholeness of silence, the silence of the Unlimited. When sound becomes audible, that profound silence is wounded and we come into being, unfolding from the heart. "The Knower" (*Prajna*), *The Mandukya Upanishad* says, is at the center of the heart in silence – it is the *bindu* and from there it unfolds and soundlessly communicates its knowing to the entire body.

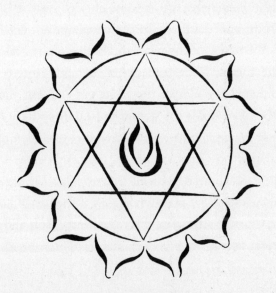

Anahata Chakra

In order to return to and know our divine and unmanifest nature we have to withdraw our awareness to the space of the heart and return to that unwounded silence. Only then are all the wounds of separation healed. Each person has to find a way of falling back into place through the space of the heart. Only from there can we hope to understand the secrets of pain, change, old age, and even death. The spirit is calling us back there constantly, but few of its calls are ones that we would consciously choose for ourselves.

Like his Indian counterpart, to the Chinese physician the heart does not simply propel the blood through the body, it also enfolds the spirit, *shen*, which suffuses every cell of our being with consciousness, making the personality of each individual an expression of this inner spirit.

The ancient Egyptians also regarded the heart as an object of awe and according to *The Egyptian Book of the Dead*, in order to cross into heaven after death you had to offer your heart to Anubis to be weighed.

What is immediately clear in these ancient systems is the fusing of the spirit and the flesh. To the people of ancient India the Divine uses the vessel of the heart to become a physical, material being. To the ancient Chinese the whole being is infused with the spiritual consciousness which the heart enfolds. For the ancient Egyptians the heart holds the account of how we have lived our lives. In these systems we are not locked away, hidden inside our heads – all that we are and have been is fully embodied.

In traditional Chinese medicine the heart is a Yin organ. Yin is the soft and yielding flow of *qi*, while Yang is the hard and resisting flow. To the Chinese physician, then, the heart is soft and yielding, even while it is strong.

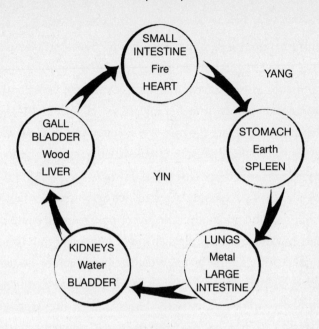

The flow of *qi*

In this ancient medical framework the vitality of each major organ of the body is said to flow from another organ which precedes it in a hierarchy. In this model the liver is the "mother" of the heart and the "child" of the kidneys.

Each organ is also assigned emotions that naturally emanate from it. The liver, *generalissimo* of the emperor heart, sees to the storage and movement of our precious vitality, determining its quantity and even flow. It is the organ that generates the emotion anger when aroused, and sustained or frequent bouts of anger can so damage the flow of vitality as to put the heart in danger.

The break-up of his marriage had sent Joe into a permanent state of anger he was unable to release except by bouts of heavy drinking in which, as a diabetic, he put his life at risk. Alcohol is an effective dampener of the liver's vitality and Joe's whole body/mind complex sought this release. To a traditional Chinese physician, Joe's diabetes would be an expected result of the environment he had created for his body. His hypertension may have been the result of excessive liver Yang, which is often associated not only with high blood pressure but also with dizziness, insomnia, and the tinnitus that Joe had first come to see me for.

Joe knew what his dreams were, but when life called upon him to adapt them he had been unable to open himself up to all the changes he was called upon to make. He was very conscious of his primary dream – to fly – and he had not let this dream go, for he was still flying and adding to it his other passion, photography. But although he had found the means and resources within himself to reorganize his life around a major change in his career, he had never allowed himself to truly open up to the pain that that had created – he had simply "got on with things" (a favorite expression of his). And then, when his divorce once again shoved him down a road he had not expected to travel, Joe had stopped going forward. Although he had had a number of relationships since the break-up of his marriage, he had not allowed anyone to get close, to get into his precious core where he could truly be touched.

Acupuncture could slowly soften Joe's hard liver Yang and coax the kidneys to yield up the precious Yin vitality that would further nourish and soften the liver. But true healing for Joe meant that he must come to terms with life's changes and arrive at a graceful reconciliation with the events that had brought him to this point in order to move on. And only Joe could do that for himself.

When Joe first started coming to see me it was clear that he had retreated into his head. His flying required clear thought and precision in acting and planning. He was engrossed in his new hobby of aerial photography that again required all kinds of detailed headwork. Joe was involving himself in all those things that did not require him to feel, just to think. But life had left two chinks in Joe's armor: his daughter and the joy of flight.

I asked Joe the question that needs asking when you are trying to open up: "How did you get here?"

This is the question that naturally follows "Where am I?" Once we have begun the process of making conscious our hidden selves, our hidden dreams, we have to explore what we have done with them and how we have arrived where we are. Joe had no problem with his basic dreams. He had flown thousands of people safely around the world many times and he was unashamed of saying that each time was a thrill. But he also freely admitted that flying himself in the small plane he had bought was far less thrilling – flying was an experience that he had to share to experience the full joy of it.

We began to look at Joe's anger. Anger can be honest, protective, and righteous, and its synergistic emotion, assertion, a great ally as we age. However, we have to find a creative and safe release for it. We have to put in place mechanisms for making it non-toxic. We may have had to swallow the poison, but like the legendary Kali we have to transform it.

Anger is too much for the body to contain indefinitely – unexpressed, it hardens into bitterness, cynicism, and depression. It broods, and its brooding always leads to violence – either directed at ourselves or others. The healing that we the aging can offer our whole community is to shatter the myth that we are by nature violent and aggressive beings and that the natural outcome of these tendencies is war.

The world-renowned anthropologist Richard Leakey argues persuasively against the idea that humans are inherently aggressive. In his book *Origins*, co-authored with Roger Lewin, Leakey looks at violence in the early human family, the hunter-gatherers, for signs of innate aggression and violence and finds no evidence for it at all:

> War is a battle for power over people and for resources such as land and minerals, neither of which are relevant in hunting and gathering societies ... One supreme biological irony underlies the entire issue of organized war in modern societies – the cooperative nature of human beings.[2]

After the breakdown of his marriage, Joe had cut himself off from people. He had encased himself in the white-hot anger that was his first response to the situation and made an unconscious decision to stay there. Anger is an acceptably male emotion and Joe did not want to open himself to any other.

In response to the question "How did you get here?" Joe himself gradually realized this and opened up to the road he was traveling. I asked him to think of the final legacy he would be giving Alice, his beloved daughter, and the children she would have – if he was lucky enough to live to meet them. I emphasized luck, explaining that if he did not change the way he was living, it was the only thing that would take him into old age.

Joe could not connect to any single person in the beginning. But he did begin to work through his anger to the emotions of pain and fear beneath it. It was a painful, sometimes even excruciating, pilgrimage.

As part of his journey towards healing and reconnecting to others, Joe began doing volunteer work with young people with learning disabilities. These people accepted him just as he was. It did not matter to them that he appeared to be grumpy – he was the man that organized for them to go up in airplanes and fly around and see their houses from the air, and for that they gave their open, uncomplicated friendship, gratitude, and love. They never knew how much healing they did for Joe, but he knew. The thrill of flying began to return because he was sharing it with others.

As he was getting to know and understand himself better, Joe's anger toward his ex-wife dissolved and his relationship with his daughter opened up to new levels of affection. His daughter was now able to feel that being happy with one parent did not mean betraying the other.

Physically, Joe's blood sugar levels, previously so out of control that it was difficult for his consultants to determine the type and dosage of insulin he needed, have now finally begun to stabilize and his tinnitus has disappeared.

Joe thinks the acupuncture is miraculous. I know he created the miracles himself by being prepared to open up and check his direction.

> The gods may well be perfect, but it seems to me that human perfection lies in not giving up.

DIEDERICK REINEKE

Returning to the Nature of The Heart

> The moral arc of the universe is long, but it bends towards justice.

REV. DR MARTIN LUTHER KING, JNR

In drawing closer to the spirit within, we pass through the *ahamkara*, the idea-of-I, and deal with the emotions of that inner instrument, of which anger is just one. When wronged, the *ahamkara* cries out for revenge, which it calls justice. But justice is found not in the philosophy of "an eye for an eye" but in the fabric of life – justice, in other words, belongs to the spirit, and working towards it has nothing to do with allowing anger to evolve into "payback." The mathematician and historian Bronowski calls this the "push-button philosophy, that is deliberately deaf to suffering and that has become the monster in the war-machine."[3]

We must be aware of the suffering – our own and that of others – and as we age we must grow in sensitivity to that suffering and lead our community towards a creative resolution of its collective anger that does not take us all down a path of assured mutual destruction. Anger in its initial phase is a *rajasic*, outward-moving, emotion. Sustained anger is tamasic, inward moving, and draws to us a darkness through which we cease to be able to see the light.

By the time Joe came to see me his anger had taken him into a deeply *tamasic* state and he was accustomed to feeling bad. He did not associate this feeling with the way he had organized himself around the events of his life. Feeling bad was what Joe had become used to and first of all he had to become acutely aware of all the feelings that were bundled together into that general "feeling bad."

Depression, anger's collaborator, has reached epidemic proportions in our society, among the aged as well as the young, and the only people benefiting from it are those with investments in pharmaceutical companies. If we adopt the "heads on sticks" approach of modern technological medicine and take the drugs they prescribe, we might become numb to our pain but its source will continue. These drugs do not only affect the cells of our brain and central nervous system. In her book *The Molecules of Emotion*, Candace Pert, a research physicist in the Department of Physiology and Biophysics at Georgetown University, points out that while the effects of modern antidepressant drugs on the brain are very precisely measured, their effects on the rest of the body and its cells are not. She describes these effects as "a cascade ... kind of like a waterfall that starts at the top but initiates changes all along the way to the bottom."[4] There are times when there is no other alternative but to be medicated, but make sure it is the last resort rather than the first. As we age we must assume full responsibility for ourselves and become informed about the choices and actions that we take, including whether or not to take medication.

> Disappointment is a good sign of basic intelligence. It cannot be compared with anything else; it is so sharp, precise, obvious and direct ... Once we open ourselves then we land on what is.

CHÖGYAM TRUNGPA[5]

Rather than seeking solace for our depression, frustration, and anger – our bundle of "feeling bad" – in drugs or alcohol as we reach middle and old age, we need to have confidence in our experience and find ways to confront these feelings and deal with them. If we do not, we will bury our soul beneath them. They are only a part of ourselves. Having matured, we have other parts that are more than equal to them.

Disappointment may lead us to what we can fulfill. Elise has finally enrolled at art school full time, after trying out some part-time courses, and that dream is no longer locked in the fabric of her body. Now her body has become her means of fulfilling it.

We Are Not the Island –
We Are the Ocean

Whatever the poet or songwriter might say, no man or woman is an island. We cannot cut ourselves off from others and expect to thrive. Many studies have now confirmed that we live longer and better when we connect with others. We are at our very best when we are giving ourselves freely. Compelling evidence exists to show that engaging our energy in work for others without any expectation of reward is one of the best ways of ensuring longevity.

Intimacy and love are as necessary for our long-term survival as food and air. In his book *Love and Survival*, the physician Dean Ornish beautifully describes the experiments in the Tecumsah Community Health Study and concludes, "Those who help others at least once a week were two and a half times less likely to die during the study as those who never volunteered. In other words, those who helped others lived longer themselves."[6]

We may not immediately be aware of the edge such giving gives us, but the ancient physicians understood clearly that it is through the altruistic connections we make with others that we become fully human.

When we do not lock away our dreams anymore or hide away from the pain of our disappointments, they are able to live in us and take us on unexpected journeys. Edna, Elise, and Joe are now all committed to being the person they were born to be. It took them to middle age to get to that kind of commitment, but they are there, finally fully aware that they are unfolding from the heart and living a life that is conscious and true to the voice of the heart. They are working to uncover the next dream that they know they embody and that they need to be present to in order to draw closer to their own True Self. None of them yearns for youth – they know where they are and have a clearer idea of how they got there, and they are working to stay open to the new changes that life will bring them.

Chapter 6

Riding the Wave
of Opening Up

Indescribable and free from motive,
Love is at the core of the internal experience.
It is subtle and yet it is profound –
When it manifests within us
We expand with it.

THE NARADA BHAKTI SUTRAS VERSE 54[1]

Once the Self unfolds from the silence of the heart to become the embodied individual, there is one profound truth that it will always seek to resonate with and that is that love is the way of creation. When we forget that ultimate truth, or let other things get in the way of it, we close down our hearts and our lives begin to resonate with that closure. When we honor love, we honor the spirit of the unburdened heart and the free flow of life.

We think of love as the emotion of the heart, but in reality love is a universal event for the body. Even our brains were built to love. In the course of our evolution from mud paddlers to apes and finally to standing, thinking humans, our brain has undergone extraordinary growth. Like some ancient city, it has grown one part upon another. On top of the ancient "reptilian brain" found in the brain stem we grew an outcropping called the cerebral cortex, a

magnificent jelly of gray matter made up of neurons and their supporting cells. The ancient brain stem carries out the vital functions
necessary for our survival, like regulating the heartbeat and respira-
tion, and acting as a relay station between the cortex and the body.
The cerebral cortex allows us to understand, perceive, remember,
communicate, and respond to the world around us. While the brain
stem can be said to represent the impulse of Earth Tattva, the will
to be, the cerebral cortex seems to better represent the impulse of
Space Tattva, the will to organize chaos into order.

Encircling the upper part of the brain stem and embraced by
the cerebral cortex is the small but mighty limbic system, the emotional part of the brain. The neuroscientist Dr Daniel Amen notes
in his book *Change Your Brain, Change Your Life*:

> The deep limbic system affects motivation and drive. It helps
> you get going in the morning and encourages you to move
> through the day ... The deep limbic structures are also intimate-
> ly involved with bonding and social connectedness.[2]

In the limbic system we find the embodiment of wind and water –
it moves us outward into contact with others and yet calls us
inward to maintain contact with ourselves.

So the brain, that seat of logic and reasoning, is also structur-
ally created to love – to touch and be touched, to reach out and to
respond. We should no more deny these impulses than the impulse
to breathe. As soon as we isolate ourselves from others and
become out of touch, we are denying what it means to be a fully
developed human with a remarkably evolved brain – and we are
closing down our heart.

What is the Heart?

In our ignorance of the True Self that is seated in the heart we have come to live in the shadow of love, and often by the time we reach middle age we have lived there for so long we mistake it for the light. Therefore, before we can begin to change our lifestyle to one that resonates with the heart and feeds it rather than starves it, we have to acknowledge the heart's deep and always urgent need to love – which is borne out by the way it serves the rest of the body.

Seated snugly in the center of the thorax, with approximately two thirds of its mass situated slightly to the left, the heart weighs less than a pound. This small organ, a hollow muscle made up of four "receiving" chambers, has a mighty job: giving blood a heave-ho on its journey through the body. While the actual walls of the heart form three layers, it is the middle layer of muscle, the myocardium, that contracts to squeeze blood into the lungs or into the rest of the body via the arteries.

The heart is divided in two: the right side receives blood that has already made the trip around the body and sends it to the lungs to pick up more oxygen and unload its excess carbon dioxide. The left side of the heart receives freshly oxygenated blood from the lungs and sends it out to the body. Because the left side has the greater job, the muscles of the left side are thicker and stronger than those of the right.

In order to sustain itself, the open loving heart needs to keep this free flow of blood to the body constant. The ways in which we close down this flow, through a diet that stifles it and a sedentary lifestyle that inhibits it, often mirror the way in which we are closing ourselves down.

We begin the process of opening up by discovering the many things that stifle love.

Walking with the Past

Following on from the previous walking meditation, when you are doing the quiet part of your walk and are all on your own, imagine you are joined by someone you have loved and who has loved you in return.

- How does it feel?

- Does your chest feel open or closed in this experience?

- Observe your gait. Does your body move more freely as you walk?

When you know the physical responses of walking with someone who loved and honored you, walk with someone who has hurt you or shamed you. Imagine the person walking right beside you. Your body will treat this image in exactly the same way it would treat the actual event. (If you doubt this, imagine that you are biting into a juicy yellow lemon and feel your saliva flow – your body has responded to an imagined event in exactly the same way it responds to it actually happening.) Let your awareness, the ever-vigilant buddhi, focus on the responses you feel in your body rather than the dialogue going on in your head.

- How does your chest feel when you walk with someone who abused your vulnerability or rejected you?

- What are the emotions that flow through your muscles and connective tissue as you walk with this person?

- Do you feel expanded or contracted?

- How does your abdomen feel?

- How tight or relaxed is your jaw?

Let your past tell your story through the sensations of your body. You will be getting to know your own mythology, the stories bound in with your past that have brought you to where you are now. Be aware of how the person who brought you pain has profoundly disturbed your feelings and how much these feelings have prevented you from being the person you want to be. Do not turn your attention from the pain, discomfort, anger, and even shame that you feel. Rather, turn and face it, and most of all feel it. Then take leave of this person and continue your walk alone.

Now speak to your feelings. Let them know you are grateful for their presence. They may have been protecting you from coming to harm, or to more harm. Tell these feelings all that you have accomplished since this pain was inflicted on you, how you have survived and maybe even triumphed in spite of that hurt. Let these feelings become your "familiars" in the old-fashioned sense of that word. It used to be believed that witches had familiars – demon spirits that were under their control. Bring these demon feelings into your open awareness and through the magical power of your attention transform them into tools that you can use to gain energy and self-understanding, rather than a button that someone else can press.

It may take only moments or it may take days or weeks or months of walking with your feelings in this way. Bring only patience, compassion, and sensitivity to the exercise.

If the person you are walking with is a person from your past, one of the influences that brought you to where you are now, ask yourself these two questions:

- "Do I wish to continue carrying these experiences in my body?"

- "How much do these physical feelings stop me being the person I want to be?"

  As you ask these questions and bring awareness to these past events, a profound sense of peace and a joy that is much deeper than pleasure will begin to grow. New perceptions will begin to fill your life because you are working at processing your experiences and integrating them into your everyday life rather than isolating them. And this, truly, is a spiritual life, one in which we become whole and integrated beings.

  If the person you were walking with is someone from your present, ask yourself the same two questions but add this question:

- "If I walk the path of the heart, what is the appropriate action to take now?"

Be very careful here. We are not called to be victims, we are called to love, and only love knows the appropriate response.

I deliberately do not advise anyone to go down the "forgiveness" path – not because I do not believe in forgiveness, but because there is so much confusion about what it involves. Sometimes we have the idea that we must allow the person we have forgiven to keep abusing us or others. Love does not make this mistake, but the confused I-maker often does. When you truly love you do not, for example, allow yourself to support the other's alcoholism or violence or any other destructive addiction or compulsion. Neither do you seek any pay-back. Offer the one you love and who has hurt you to the forces of life, let life take care of them. And do for yourself what love tells you to do: step out free and move on.

There might be several people from your past waiting for your

attention. This is the way we find out how we got here. All these people have brought you to where you are now. But the person you have
become is greater than any single one of them. You will find that you
have made yourself out of those experiences, but the self that you are
is also the miracle that those experiences produced, even when the
experiences themselves were filled with trauma.

It may help to write down your experiences with your walking
meditation when you get home and keep a journal of this part of
your journey.

Narrowing the Flow

Like all other muscles the heart needs blood to keep functioning
and any obstruction in the flow will cause the muscle to stop
working. We call this a heart attack (myocardial infarction).
Depending on how much muscle is affected, the heart attack will
either be severe enough to kill or mild enough to cause hospitaliza-
tion and a radical review of lifestyle.

Restrictions in blood flow to the heart can be caused by
atherosclerosis. Atherosclerosis is when the arteries – the network
of rivers that carry oxygen-rich blood from the heart to the tissues
of the body – become simultaneously hardened, inflexible, and
clogged. The actual wall of the artery thickens and intrudes into
the space where blood should be flowing. If this happens in one
of the arteries to the heart, it causes a heart attack; if it happens in
one of the arteries to the brain, it causes a stroke.

The main culprit in atherosclerosis is cholesterol. Yet far from
being a dragon come to slay us in youth, cholesterol is a fatty substance that provides the structural basis for all our natural steroids
as well as the outer lining of our cells. Our body manufactures

cholesterol in the liver and then organizes a complicated delivery system via the bloodstream to get it to the cells where it is needed. However, another source of cholesterol is our diet. Meals that contain flesh, fish, and fowl all have a high cholesterol content. Once the body has ingested this cholesterol it is absorbed into the blood. After a heavy, high-cholesterol meal, the hard-working liver will remove these cholesterol particles from the blood and in between meals manufacture cholesterol to put back into the bloodstream.

Cholesterol is carried around our bloodstream by tiny round bodies called lipoproteins. Low density lipoproteins (LDLs) pick up a large packet of cholesterol and a small amount of protein and head off via the arteries to deliver their cargo to the cells of the body. If they do not find a proper site to deliver the cholesterol to they simply dump their load in the arteries, where it begins to clump together around the walls, forming a hard, thick plaque. After a while, as this plaque thickens, it begins to obstruct the free flow of blood, thus reducing the blood and oxygen supply to the body.

Being kind, nature evolved a solution to the problem. Other lipoproteins, called high density lipoproteins (HDLs), which carry less cholesterol and more protein, run around picking up the cholesterol from the bloodstream that has not successfully been delivered to cells by the LDLs and carry it back to the liver.

However, to remove cholesterol from the blood the liver relies on special receptors on the surface of its cells which snatch the cholesterol particles from the blood flowing through it and then transport it into its interior. A fast removal of LDL cholesterol means you have a high number of LDL receptors in your liver. If you have a high cholesterol level it might mean that you are low in LDL receptors in the liver.

Diets high in saturated fats (derived mostly from meat and dairy products) decrease LDL receptor activity. Changing your lifestyle to take in more fiber, fruit and vegetables (which contain no cholesterol), and exercising more can actually increase your LDL receptor activity. Unsaturated fats (like non-hydrogenated vegetable oils) can sometimes even lower cholesterol levels, particularly oils like extra virgin pressed olive oil or cold-pressed flax seed oil.

Hearts, Fats, and the Spirit

Our lifeblood should flow freely from the heart throughout the body, just as the spirit flows from the *bindu* to become mind, breath, and body. Obstructions in our arteries are often a mirror of the obstructions we are placing in the way of our spiritual unfolding, obstructions like anger and its siblings bitterness, depression, and cynicism. It is hard to connect with a good lifestyle that will keep the heart healthy and the blood in free flow when these emotions are blocking our path. It is difficult to distance oneself from these emotions and view them objectively, but try this exercise next time you find yourself becoming angry.

Overcoming Anger

This is a difficult emotion to deal with because, like fear, it is often a protecting emotion.

- First of all acknowledge that your anger may be quite justified and absolutely righteous. Anger is not in itself bad – it is, after all, a manifestation of Fire Tattva that provides energy and passion.

- Now ask yourself, "What is my anger bringing to this particular situation?" Anger may not be justified; it can simply be our habitual response to certain situations and then we risk it contaminating other-wise loving relationships.

The way to handle anger is not through suppression but through acknowledgment and awareness. Once you have become accus-tomed to working with the awareness using the exercises in the previ-ous chapter, you can use this meditation to deal with anger:

- If you are in the white-hot throes of anger, immediately remove yourself from the situation. Go somewhere where you can be alone for just a few moments. Pace up and down or stamp your feet a few times if these physical activities will help discharge the build-up of energy, and then sink into the awareness.

- There is awareness and there is anger. Both exist simultaneously. Move your position from the anger into the awareness.

- Let more and more of yourself slide into the awareness. Become aware of the breath and focus on the out-breath in particular. Breathe out through the nose and let your out-breath slow down.

- Focus your attention on the stillpoint between breaths. After a while feel that you are drawing your presence from the circle of anger until you are entirely situated in the circle of awareness.

- Become aware of where in your body you feel the anger, where it is physically situated.

- Begin to breathe into that physical place. Continue to breathe out much more slowly than you breathe in. Engage the abdominal muscles to complete the exhalation. Let the awareness and the breath begin to transform the immediacy of the anger.

- Only go back into the situation when you are firmly established in the awareness and your body feels that it is organizing itself differently around the experience of anger.

Dr Daniel G. Amen suggests in his book *Change Your Brain, Change Your Life* that the left temporal lobe of the cerebral cortex is our "anger" center and that we can calm down this area by chanting long vowel sounds like aaaaah (known as toning) or by gentle humming. If you have a problem with anger, why not make some time each day for some gentle toning and humming?

The Meditation of Silence

The heart, an expression of Anahata Chakra, is renewed by silence. Make some time for yourself during the week when all radios, telephones, and televisions are switched off. Silence the space you have control over. Let what you have no control over fall into the silence of your heart using this meditation.

- Sit in a comfortable chair or posture in which your back, neck, and head easily flow in a straight line.

- Feel your contact with the support beneath you at your sitting bones, legs, and feet, and let your weight flow down through your body, through these points of contact, into the support beneath you.

- With each exhalation release more and more weight, freeing your spine to flow up. Feel your head balancing on the crown of the spine.

- Follow the out-breath to the stillpoint between breaths and let your attention become focused on that point, watching for the very first movement that gives rise to the next breath, watching intently to find the source of each in-breath.

- Now become aware of what you are hearing, of all of the sounds entering the room from the outside and any sounds inside, screening out nothing.

- Keep listening intently.

- Gradually become aware of the place in your head where you hear
  these sounds – your listening point.

- Move your awareness from the sounds themselves to the point, the
  focus of hearing.

- Slowly and deliberately draw this focus of hearing down into the base
  of your throat. Feel now that all sound is heard in the base of the throat.

- Keep the point of listening established there for a while.

- Slowly and deliberately draw the focus of listening down again, this
  time into the center of your heart. Feel that you are listening to the
  world from the cave of your heart.

- Gradually feel that these sounds are entering a space of vast silence, a
  silence so powerful that it absorbs all sound into its silence.

- Stay established in that silence for some time.

- Then gradually become aware of the whole of your body and personality evolving from this silence, unfolding from this center.

- Complete your meditation by standing up and stretching out, opening
  your arms wide and letting the vitality of your heart flow out through
  your fingertips.

As you begin to reconnect to the spirit of your heart through these
exercises you can also begin to adopt practices of exercise and diet
that will strengthen and protect your heart.

Strengthening the Heart

Like any other muscle the heart needs a regular workout to stay in good shape. We can maintain and even increase its strength by means of a regular cardiovascular workout routine. Remember that working with the body is part of the spiritual journey. The body has unfolded from the spirit, the Self of the heart – there is no duality, they are one.

Every cell in your body burns sugars in the presence of oxygen to produce energy – the vital component of loving, giving, and living a life. The cells receive oxygen and nutrition – including the sugars they burn – from the blood being pumped through the arteries by the heart. Different parts of our body need more oxygen and nutrients than others – the brain, for instance, uses massive amounts of oxygen, as do the muscles that make us move, including the heart.

A problem arises when we become sedentary and the heart muscle grows weak. Then the muscles of the body waste away and the heart has to work hard to supply the body. Added to this is the fact that a sedentary lifestyle promotes atherosclerosis, especially if it accompanies poor eating habits. A good cardiovascular routine in which the big muscles of the legs and buttocks and the muscles of the arms are being used means that the body will begin to create miles of new arteries to feed these hard-working muscles, reducing the amount of work the heart has to do to get the blood to the body. Regular exercise also stimulates receptor sites on the surface of the liver cells to absorb the LDLs that would otherwise be dumping their load of cholesterol in the arteries.

Aerobic exercise is what you are aiming for. Aerobic simply means "with oxygen." Aerobic exercise uses stored fat to fuel the muscles rather than drawing on glucose from the liver (which is what happens in anaerobic exercise). It can be running, walking briskly, or any other activity that uses the muscles of the legs, and if possible arms, so that you start breathing more deeply and the heart starts sending the blood coursing through the body. Exercise stops being aerobic when you are panting and unable to carry out a conversation.

By careful monitoring you can devise a system that is both aerobic and enjoyable – joy is the positive emotion of the heart, so let your routine be a joyful experience! My own favorite is dancing. Really rock, ensuring that you include some jumping around, and sustain it all for 30 minutes three or four times a week. My body and my heart remember the joy and exuberance of youth and bring it back into my life each time I do this. In his book *Ageless Body, Timeless Mind*, Dr Deepak Chopra recounts an experiment conducted at Harvard University in 1979 in which a group of people were put in an environment that perfectly reflected 1959 and were asked to relate to each other as if it were 1959 and they were young again. At the end of the experiment various biological measurements showed a dramatic improvement in health and reversal in aging, proving that "so-called irreversible signs of aging could be reversed using psychological intervention."[3] No wonder I feel so peppy after a 30-minute session of wild dancing to Jimi Hendrix or the Mamas and the Papas, two of my favorites from my teens and early twenties!

Whether you are using walking, running, or dancing, when you begin this program take your pulse for a full minute in the morning before you get out of bed and write it down. You will discover that after a few months of doing your cardiovascular workout your resting pulse rate comes down a few notches – this is a sign that your cardiovascular system is growing stronger. The heart muscle has strengthened and the arteries are more receptive, so the heart does not have to work so hard and fast to send blood to the body.

A Lifestyle of Non-violence

Ahimsa, the practice of living life in such a way that we do no harm or violence to others, has long attracted people from all walks of life and traditions. Made popular in the last century by Mahatma Gandhi and the Rev. Dr Martin Luther King, Jnr, it is a way of living that seems in harmony with the way of the heart.

Once you have committed yourself to the life of the heart, a life of love and joy for this second half of your life, you will want to change your lifestyle to bring life to the heart. Heart disease is the number one killer in all Western technologically sophisticated societies and the primary cause of heart disease is still smoking. Smoking is one of the most pervasive forms of violence we do to ourselves, and as long as we continue we cannot hope to live a life of non-violence towards others. Breath – oxygen – is life. Drawing into your body substances that will harm rather than give life is a commitment to a slow suicide. If you are still caught in the vicious trap of this highly addictive substance, one that would not get past our food and drug administrations were it introduced now, question that commitment with each puff. It's not cool to smoke – it's turning your lungs black and furring up your arteries and depriving your body of oxygen, and it is aging you more rapidly than the birthdays that are coming around each year.

The next thing to look at is your diet. Anyone still eating a non-vegetarian diet has not fully opened their heart and properly understood the violence we do to other beings that share this planet with us when we deliberately breed and feed them to kill them. Ask yourself, "Is this the life of the heart?"

If only from a sense of enlightened self-interest you should take a careful look at your diet in terms of saturated fats – all animal fats are saturated fats.

Always evaluating how your action will affect others may help, perhaps using the Gandhi maxim: "Before you take any action ask yourself how this action will affect the poorest, the most voiceless on the planet." In this regard it is helpful to know that 70 per cent of all cultivated crops on this planet are fed to animals that we in turn kill to eat. In his highly informative book *Diet for a New America*, John Robbins points out that: "The world's cattle alone, not to mention pigs and chickens, consume a quantity of food equal to the caloric needs of 8.7 billion people – nearly double the entire human population of the planet."[4] By changing our diet to conform to the flow of the heart, we could wipe out starvation on Earth.

As you engage in these practices and open up to the life of the heart, you will encounter those dreams and hopes that can no longer be fulfilled, and you will find the strength to let them go and let love flow where anger, disappointment, and bitterness were settling in.

Only the unburdened heart opens itself up as a pathway back to the infinite, back to our own true nature, turning towards the mystery of eternity and away from the myth of mortality, which is all the ahamkara knows.

As you allow yourself to make the changes that are necessary, you must enter the next wave, the wave of Staying in Touch.

The Third Wave

Chapter 7

Stay in Touch

Each of us arrives into this world with various needs. One of these is the need for touch ... regardless of how much the intensity of the touch varies, the need remains. Touch is not simply a pleasant stimulus but a biological necessity.

PHYLLIS K. DAVIS[1]

As we call upon long-forgotten dreams and retrieve buried pain in order to remain open to this human spiritual journey, we come to a wave that influences all the others. It is the wave that requires that we

Stay in Touch.

To age with spirit we must stay in touch both with ourselves and with others. We do this through the practices we are already engaged in and by embracing new habits that will ensure that we keep attuned to the receding shoreline on which the children and grandchildren of our generation still live.

Our spiritual practices cannot be divorced from the lives we are leading. To realize the True Self as we age, and to begin to identify more and more deeply with it, without doubt or fear, we have to involve consciousness and life. We cannot forsake one to grow strong in the other. With bodies that are aging we still have to engage in life, but from a spiritual dimension – a dimension of consciousness. On this journey we leave behind that artificial separation of spirit and body that we have grown up with, and we accept the life of the body as a reflection of the spirit and allow it to be our guide. After all, not only is the body the thing we are most familiar with, it is also the closest to hand!

Alone Among Many

On reaching her fifties Maureen had begun to suffer from mild memory loss – silly things like not remembering where she had left her keys or being unable to remember a name when introduced to someone new. Quite naturally she became worried that this presaged that dreaded monster of aging, dementia. After banks of tests her doctor was able to reassure her that she was probably suffering from nothing more than mild anxiety and recommended she try Yoga as a means of relaxation rather than medication. Her first Yoga teacher was a sensitive woman, deeply committed to both the spiritual and physical aspects of Yoga, and Maureen, who had been born into the Church of England but never been a churchgoer, felt drawn to the spiritual practices she was being put in touch with. Soon she was going on weekend retreats to learn more about meditation and crafting regular times to meditate into her day as she became more fully in touch with the spiritual side of her nature that had been silently waiting for her attention.

When I met Maureen and she told me her personal story I was deeply moved by her ability to put herself last on her list of priorities. She was married to a barrister and had a daughter who was following in her father's footsteps. The entire household was organized around the needs of the careers of her husband and daughter and Maureen had been reduced to the status of service provider with very little personal contact with either of them. She told me they had not noticed when she no longer joined them for evening meals after she had cooked and set the meal out for them. She related all this in a jolly voice, triumphant that they did not notice when she slipped away for hours or weekends to further her spiritual studies as long as she ensured that the household ran smoothly for them while she was away. Amidst this isolation she had withdrawn into a world of meditation and prayerful chanting. And her forgetfulness persisted. I was also aware that after five years of Yoga her body still appeared stiff and unyielding.

Maureen's isolation is by no means unusual. Throughout the Western world there are conscientious middle-aged women and men who have provided mindfully and with loving care for their families but whose needs and cares have been set aside by those they have provided for. It is then all too easy to accept this imposed isolation and find compensation in "spirituality." But our spiritual nature is too important to be assigned the role of compensator – it seeks always to be balanced and expressed through the way we live our lives. Through our senses, and most particularly through our sense of touch, the spirit teaches us that isolation is not the answer.

The Self at the Surface

The spirit that forms the cells of the human body in order to manifest itself creates a profound sense of touch very early in the development of the fetus. Receptors that will have extraordinary

sensitivity for measuring internal and external touch develop earlier
than any other senses. From then on, just as the blind touching
raised paper are able to distinguish letters and words, we will use
this sense of touch to "see." In fact, in one way or another, all the
other senses mimic this one remarkable sense. And while seeing,
hearing, tasting, and smelling are confined to the area of the head
and face, touch is universal throughout the body. It is as if the Self
is emerging at the surface of our being to make contact with everything that the I-maker considers "other."

Each of the five chakras is associated with one of the senses.
Touch is associated with Anahata Chakra, the heart. In the previous chapter we looked at that aspect of Anahata which embraces
the Self extending through the body in the tide of our circulation.
But Vayu Tattva, the Air element, moves across the Earth's surface,
sending clouds scurrying through the sky, rousing the sea, and fanning fires to make them rage out of control, and it does all of this in
us also. It moves the other tattvas into a rajasic state and it is most
fully expressed in the body through the nervous system, the major
communication system of the body.

Signals run through the body along nerve fibers and leap over
synapses, instructing muscles to contract, heads to spin, sensations
to enter. Hormones and neurotransmitters, also communicators,
wash through the body's oceans at a more leisurely pace, bumping
into the surfaces of cells until they find synchronous receptors that
perfectly understand their message and relay it into the heart of the
cell. Without these sophisticated communication systems we
would be immobilized – our lungs would cease to breathe, our
hearts would cease to beat, our minds would cease to think. So
important is this capacity for communication that life seems to
have made it a universal event not confined to nerves, synapses,
hormones, and receptors. Remember the sperm cells in the petri

dish that continued to communicate with the body they had come from, even when it was 40 feet away? Such communication seems to know no barriers – neither empty space nor solid walls. It demands that the buddhi continues to expand beyond the boundary of our skin to seek out all that there is.

Inside Out

> The skin is no more separated from the brain than the surface of a lake is separated from its depths; the two are different locations in a continuous medium ... To touch the surface is to stir the depth.
>
> DEANE JUHAN[2]

As we saw with the first wave, Making the Unconscious Conscious, all tissue in the body is formed from just three simple layers of cells: the mesoderm, the ectoderm, and the endoderm. Before the first month of pregnancy has passed, a raised groove appears on the back of the embryo, marking a longitudinal line down its length. This is known as the "primitive streak." As soon as it appears, the ectoderm cells begin a frenzy of activity that involves both migration and transformation. Using the primitive streak as their marker, they loop and fold to create a groove that will eventually form the neural canal and central nervous system of the body. As if this is not remarkable enough, in the process of looping and folding to become the brain and spinal cord, the ectoderm also becomes our outermost skin! Thus that which holds the entire store of our knowledge – the record of our lives – extends outwards to become our boundary in touch with the world. The internal and external are integral to each other.

The design of the nervous system is breathtakingly complex.

We simplify it for discussion and study, and because the ahamkara needs to separate and categorize in order to understand. Thus the completely whole and integrated nervous system is artificially divided into the central and peripheral "systems."

The central nervous system is that part which is contained within the spine and skull, and the peripheral nervous system is all the nerve tissue outside it. Via these two systems messages flow between the brain and the body at breakneck speeds. These messages tell us to reach out and touch or to retreat from danger, to change course, to continue – all the million and one things each of us does in the course of a day. Right now, touch receptors distributed throughout your body are relaying messages via your nervous system about the touch of clothes against your skin; keeping your brain in constant touch with the support beneath you, whether you are standing, sitting, or lying down; monitoring the touch of air against your skin and even within your nose, throat, and lungs; giving and receiving information about how much effort is needed to hold the weight of this book, and so on.

The cells of the nervous system have extraordinary longevity – they are able to survive for over 100 years. This is just as well because, like the cells of the heart muscle, nerve cells are not replaceable – they do not multiply by endless division. Nerve cells are also hungry: they have an extremely high metabolic rate and demand a constant supply of oxygen and glucose. Thus the brain gets between seven and nine times more blood than any other organ.

Situated in the brain, nerve cells called neurons have large cell bodies that are the factories where information coming in from the senses is dealt with. Reaching out from this cell body is a network of extensions called dendrites that grow outcroppings like seaweed, fanning out to be in touch with the dendrites of other neurons and creating a brain that resembles an underwater forest of seaweed so thick that one branch can barely be distinguished from another. Like exquisitely crafted lace, dendrites connect to one another to receive the information that they convey back to the body of the neuron. Each neuron also sends out a long slender tail called an axon that reaches down into the spinal cord and from there into the body. We call these axons nerve fibers. Through these dendrites and axons information is passed between neurons and the body. It is through these extensions that the brain stays in touch with the internal environment of the body and the external environment that it is living in.

Our brain, as we see from these "systems," is not isolated from our body – whatever feeds or deprives the body will nourish or starve the brain. And our brain needs us to stay in touch – in all the ways that it is possible for us to do so. Messages to and from the brain are carried on nerve fibers in an electrical current, but unlike any other electrical current, a nerve impulse continually regenerates itself along the entire length of the extension of the nerve cell so that its message does not deteriorate with distance. And all of this happens without our conscious input at speeds as great as 120 miles per second.

As we age, the brain begins to suffer the loss of some nerve cells. The visual cortex at the back of the brain that governs our sight and the sensory parts at the sides are the most affected. But no matter how old we get, nerve cells demonstrate both a willingness and a capacity to create new connections to partner other nerve cells. If, as many scientists believe, this is the basis for learning, it appears that our nervous system remains ever ready for new lessons. Old dogs can indeed learn new tricks. As we enter middle age we have to grasp this capacity and work with it, not isolate and deprive ourselves. Denying the impulses of wind and fire by retreating from the world will only hasten the withdrawal of vitality from these spheres of the body.

> ... recent research suggests that certain cortical neurons seem actually to become more abundant after maturity has been reached, and these cells reside in precisely the areas in which the processes of higher thought take place ... neuroscientists may actually have discovered the source of the wisdom which we like to think we can accumulate with advancing age.
>
> SHERWIN B. NULAND[3]

So, though we lose brain cells as we age, it seems that provided we can walk the path nature has chalked for us, we can still live and learn. But to do so, like a neuron reaching out into the world of light and dark, heat and cold, good and bad, from the protection of the skull and spine, we need to reach out and stay in touch.

When Edna, Elise, Joe, and Maureen began to confront the ways in which they were closing themselves down they had a clear choice: they could continue with their lives on exactly the same trajectory or they could change direction. Once you have asked the questions "Where am I?" and "How did I get here?", the next question is: "Where am I going?" If you project yourself forward into the future, with all your current habits of thinking and doing, what landscape do you see? Does your current way of life support a future that is in touch with, still in love with, the world around you?

Remember, we are created to love and to continue loving, and to learn and to continue learning. Just as the brain is in touch with the rest of the body, so we have to stay in touch with life. Discovery is the impulse of the Self that created a nervous system working at speeds faster than lightning striking the ground. We have to overcome a psychology that tells us that once we have passed a certain age we can no longer change, and embrace the wisdom of the body that is in a constant state of change and renewal.

Retreating and losing touch with those she loved was beginning to have its effect on Maureen through low-key anxiety, and she had to re-evaluate her environment. She had to get in touch with herself as a whole rather than as fragments labeled "wife," "mother," and "spiritual aspirant." Using some of the exercises from the previous chapters and from the next, she began to remember all that she was. She recalled the joy she once had when teaching signing to deaf children and she understood enough about herself to know that she wanted to live a life giving to others. Providing for a family had been one way of fulfilling this need, but as she lost touch with those she was providing for, it ceased to be creative or fulfilling. Her husband remained unapproachable on the subject of their partnership and often became patronizing when she tried to discuss it, pointing out that many women envied the lifestyle he had provided for her.

One day Maureen left home. Having made all the arrangements, she told her shocked husband and daughter, who had just sat down to the evening meal she had prepared, that while she still loved them deeply, she was taking time out and leaving for South America to work with deaf and dumb children and that she did not know how long she would be away. Then she turned round, walked out to the waiting taxi, and left for the airport.

She is still in South America, working with abandoned children. A few months ago I received an e-mail from her that was full of joy and showed none of the "muddle-headedness" that she had earlier accused herself of. She said that her husband wanted her to return home, but that she did not yet feel strong enough in her own purpose not to lose herself in his indifference, which she thought might re-emerge as the routine of their days together was re-established.

Maureen is learning about the world – the world of her family and the world outside it – and she is also learning about herself. The key that made her change direction was the question "Where am I going?" When she projected herself forward 10 or 15 years she saw a barren landscape not only for herself but also for her husband, and knew if they were to recover the respect and intimacy they had once shared they needed to reassess their views of each other. Maureen still serves, but now she is deeply engaged with those she is serving and they with her. She is also trying to find a way back to her family – a way that is wholesome and loving. She still meditates and prays, but now these practices are a fulfillment, not an escape.

Desire – The Impulse of the Soul

As profound as touch is, it is also the most censored of all our senses and in our Western society has now become almost entirely confined to sex. Yet touch is the only way we can know the sharpness of the wind or the softness of a baby's skin. And even the touch of sensuality can lead us to the spirit. As we age we retreat behind our wrinkling skin, afraid that our touch may repulse – as if touch were created only for dewy-complexioned youth. This fear often isolates us from our own sensuality and it is all too easy then to retreat into spirituality and forget the ground, the body that so perfectly expresses the spirit.

As we age we may choose to be celibate or find ourselves compelled to celibacy by the loss of a partner. On the other hand

we may be in a position to continue an active sex life and to celebrate our sexuality. Whatever our situation, we should never deny
the power of our sexual vitality that flows from Apas Tattva, the
Water element, giving us the gift to create. Whether we engage in
sex or not, remaining present to our sexuality and all the vitality
associated with it keeps us open, in touch, vulnerable, and ready to
experience the joy of the spirit and to co-operate with the spirit in
the act of creation. To do this we must work against social impera-
tives that seek to isolate us from our own bodies, just as they seek
to isolate the aging from the young.

Because sex is our means of procreation, aging often gives rise
to the myth that once procreation is no longer possible, sex is
unnecessary. As we age we have to reclaim our sexual vitality, and
by recognizing its potency within ourselves allow it equal sover-
eignty with our thinking and emotional processes.

The essential teaching of the Divine as the spirit of sensuality
is beautifully depicted in scenes of lovemaking among the gods on
one of the temple walls at Khajuraho, India. The extraordinary
grace and symmetry of this temple complex, built during the 10th
and 11th centuries, offers us a way of reconciling the divine and
the sensual in our nature. Kandariya Mahadeo, one of the temples
of this complex, rises up from the earth in raw and awe-inspiring
beauty as if sculpted by the forces of nature rather than crafted by
human hands. It stands as a testimony to human embodiment of
the Divine in all of our activities. On the temple walls, gods and
goddesses embrace in erotic love play and various stages of sexual
intercourse, symbolizing the coming together of matter and spirit.
Here sex is solemn ritual, able to lift the viewer outside a destructive philosophy in which body and spirit are required to engage
in separate and opposite pursuits to find fulfillment. What the
great rishis who inspired this temple building understood was that

human beings must engage in life as a means of expressing the spirit.

Desire is a part of what it is to be human, and in the 129th hymn of the tenth book of the Rig Veda, it is part of what it means to be divine:

Neither existence nor non-existence,
Neither space nor sky then.
What covered all?
What sheltered all?
What concealed all?
Was it water with its bottomless abyss?

There was not death
Yet there was no immortality.
There was no time between day and night.
Only the One was,
Breathing Breathless by Itself.
Beyond That – nothing.

Darkness upon darkness,
An ocean without light –
The life-force lay still,
Covered by the husk of nothingness.
Then it burst forth,
One nature from the intense heat.

Desire came upon it
And with that came the beginning –
That was the seed of the mind.
Only singers in their hearts discern
This bond between created things
And the Great Uncreate.

Kandariya Mahadeo is a monument to the simultaneous engagement of consciousness and action being the totality of creation. We
engage in life even while we stay conscious of an inner sense, a
presence that is beyond this material existence and which belongs
to eternity.

"Don't Touch!" – The Body Dislocated

> ... muscular stiffness, limitation of movement, tiredness, distor-
> tion of posture, and chronic pain are misinterpreted as the
> effects of "old age" – a fictitious disease ... In fact, however, age
> has nothing to do with it. These events are the result of an
> accumulation of physiological reactions to stress ...

THOMAS HANNA[4]

When I was a child in Africa we used to enjoy playing with fat
brown worms called shongalolas. In response to our touch the
shongalola would wrap itself into a perfect tight circle. Humans
respond in much the same way when startled. In response to any
sudden loud noise or threatening event, a cascade of neuronal signals sends our bodies into what is called the "startle reflex." The
muscles in our face and jaw tighten, our shoulders come up, our
chin juts out and muscles at the back of the neck shorten, simultaneously our abdomen tightens and the lower back pulls upward as
the knees come forward, placing us in a position that resembles a
crouch. This response is much more primitive than our voluntary
movements, and much, much faster. Strangely, it is the posture that
we have most come to associate with aging.

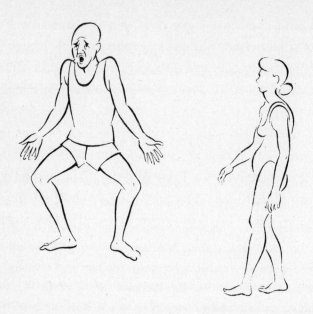

The startle reflex and the posture of "old age"

Thomas Hanna, the founder of Somatics, a form of bodywork that seeks to restore movement and flexibility, notes that many people today are fixed in this posture, or parts of it. The harmful consequences of this posture for our general health, including our digestion, circulation, and sexual functioning, have been noted by several bodyworkers. As a Yoga teacher I have come to notice how prevalent this posture is, even in people in their twenties and thirties. Very often those who have this posture complain about similar problems – depression, sleeplessness, poor digestion, constipation, loss of sexual desire, and impotence.

By its very nature the startle reflex isolates – it is meant to in order to isolate us from danger. Pain also isolates. If it is a pain of the body, we isolate that area and organize our movements around it to protect it. If it is an emotional pain, we isolate those feelings and organize our emotional lives around them. To stop organizing ourselves around our pain and isolation means we have to confront the ways in which we are isolating our thoughts and our emotions – and using our bodies to maintain that isolation.

Tragically, we can become isolated by the pettiest things as easily as we can by the big things. A couple locked in combat in which war never breaks out but hostilities are kept simmering, a parent demanding of adult children that they still conform to the parent's way of doing things, neighbors refusing to negotiate with each other over easily resolved matters, these are some of the ways in which we keep ourselves out of touch with each other and keep the world at war. To have peace we have to work for peace with as much commitment as we work to defend ourselves. That means releasing ourselves physically, emotionally, and psychologically from the startle reflex and a state of readiness for hostilities, and opening ourselves up to being in touch.

The Stillness of Being

In our hearts, the awareness, the buddhi that holds the reins of the I-maker, is speaking in a soft whisper and praying for release from the tyranny of doing into the stillness of being. Only in that stillness can we discover the ways in which we have lost touch and how we can get back in touch. As we start out on that road the heart is asking the question "Where are you going?"

By the time we reach middle age we have an urgent need to clarify the answer to that question. We may have arrived where we are now by dint of circumstances that were so difficult they were almost impossible to confront while they were happening. But we have to make the time and space in our lives now to simply be, and to contemplate our direction.

We sometimes reach middle and old age needing to relearn how to connect, how to get past pain, anger, and disappointment, and relive the experience of touching deeply and affectionately. We need to muster the resources and the lessons of a lively nervous system powered by Vayu Tattva – the Air that moves and drives. If we reach middle age and our family or friends cease to be the people with whom we are still deeply connected, we need to open up our circle and seek out new connections. Keeping in touch is about seeing who we are in relation to the world around us and not accepting isolation from it any more than the brain accepts isolation from the body.

When we truly unfold from the heart, the body shows no signs of withdrawing from the world – it reaches out and our sense of touch sustains a vision of ourselves as whole and yet part of a greater whole.

Chapter 8

Riding the Wave
of Staying in Touch

For most of us, losing our minds, dementia, is high on the list of fears associated with aging. Memory makes each of us unique – after all, it is the store of our individual life experiences. The fact is that while we may lose irreplaceable neurons as we age, neuroscience now knows that the brain continues to be extraordinarily plastic and malleable. Recent research has shown that exercising the brain spurs the growth of new extensions from neurons in order to make new connections even in very old age.

In 1994, the remarkable nuns of Mankato, Minnesota, made it into *Life* magazine. In this small community of 150 retired nuns, 25 are older than 90. Their community is drawn from a cross-section of the US, so their longevity cannot be traced to genes. Not only do these Sisters of Notre Dame live much longer than the average American, they retain remarkable cognitive functions well into old age. One of the nuns whose story was covered by the magazine, Sister Marcella, only stopped teaching formally at the age of 97, and then still kept the other nuns on their intellectual toes by doing quizzes and playing word-games with them. So remarkable is the sisters' achievement that they have been persuaded to contribute their brains to medical research on their death.

Inspired by them and the older people we all have known in our lifetime, let us find a way of riding this wave that will keep us in touch with ourselves and the world and yet on the path of the spirit.

Memory – Use It or Lose It

When the brain is compared to a computer with words like "input" and "retrieval," it's easy to get the impression that we store events in a precise and orderly manner that exactly replicates the information received from the outside. But just think of five people witnessing the same accident – each of them will store the memory in a very different way. And even if the broad details are similar in the retelling, there will be variations.

The amount of research that has gone into the way that we store memories could fill libraries, and yet much of it remains a mystery. We do know that memory is a holistic event involving interaction of almost the entire brain and body – masses of information is flowing in through the senses to the sensory area of the cortex to become two parallel circuits that involve the entire globe of the brain.

Memory involves two distinct stages: short term and long term. Short-term memory captures the fleeting event of sensory information flowing in front of you and it can last for a few seconds or a few hours. It is limited in its capacity to a few chunks of information, like a telephone number or a conversation. Long-term memory, on the other hand, seems to have an infinite capacity. Our short-term memory may not be able to recall a name it heard an hour ago, but our long-term memory not only recalls scores of names, faces, addresses, and birthdays associated with those names, but also preferences in foods that go with those names, our relations with them, what pets they have, what their hobbies are, and even their favorite colors.

Information from the senses floods into our cerebral cortex and is then selected for short-term or long-term memory. Some information that is initially placed in short-term memory will be transferred to the long term. This transfer is dependent on a number of factors:

- Emotion: Information received in a highly emotional state is always sent into long-term memory – that is how so many of us remember where we were and what we were doing when events like the September 11th attack on the World Trade Center occurred.
- Repetition: If information is repeated often enough it will eventually be stored in long-term memory.
- Association: If "new" information is associated with or relates to "old" information, it will more easily be stored in long-term memory.
- Automatic memory: Sensory information like the smell surrounding an event or the color of a book you were learning from will automatically be part of the memory.

Making a spiritual journey requires all of our cognitive functions to be as sharp as possible. In my years of spiritual work I have gone out of my way to meet great spiritual teachers from diverse traditions, and what struck me about all of them is how absolutely sharp their minds were, regardless of their age. These women and men, while embracing wholly the life of the spirit, kept their minds alive and inquiring.

As with all things, it seems the more we use our brain, the healthier and stronger it remains. And as we age there are a number of things we want to retain – our memory and our capacity to learn and reason probably being at the top of the list.

Memory Exercise 1: Memorize

Take an author you find particularly inspirational and decide to commit to memory a verse, a paragraph, or a half page of their work each
day. Decide how much time you are going to allot to this activity.
Rather than giving a half hour and then nothing more till the next day,
research has suggested that breaking up the learning session and
associating the information with previous information or other sensory
input will assist in the learning process. Remember, the achievement
here is not just learning the verse, it's learning how your brain best
remembers things so that you know how to get the most out of it as
you grow older. Try these simple variations:

- Learn for 10 or 15 minutes and then put the book down; return to it
  after two hours and give it another 10 minutes, and then return after a
  lapse of about five or six hours.

- Put the book on a piece of brightly colored cloth so that you associate
  what you are learning with the color. Change the color when you are
  learning from a new chapter or a new book.

- Burn some essential oils during your learning session. High up our nose,
  level with our eyebrows and no bigger than a thumbnail, are the smell
  receptors called the olfactory epithelia. The different smells that we
  breathe in arrive as chemical signals at this juncture and are translated
  into electrical signals that rapidly find their way straight into the cerebral
  cortex, hippocampus, and limbic system of the brain – all places active
  in the storing of memory. By associating your verses with a smell, you
  are 'burning' the memory in quicker and when you again smell that
  scent those verses will come to mind. (When I had a cold once I put
  some drops of eucalyptus oil on my pillow as I lay in bed reading the
  Catholic mystic Thomas Merton. A couple of years later I put some
  drops of eucalyptus oil in a hot bath and as the smell hit my nose these
  words drifted through my consciousness: "Our salvation begins on the

level of common and natural and ordinary things ..." I only recalled where and when I had read those words when I was lying back soaking in the bathtub, but I was profoundly impressed by olfactory senses that could so stimulate my memory as to bring back words read long ago.)

- Play some music while you are learning. Bach and Mozart, they say, increase our intellectual capacities while we listen to them. My own experience is that the drone of Tibetan monks chanting or the sweet sound of women's voices singing the famous Gregorian chants or the music of Eric Clapton do the same thing. Find music that works for you.

Memory Exercise 2: Make New Memories

Stimulate your nervous system to make new memories. If there is a car or train journey you have to take regularly, change it in some way. Take a different route, change at different stations. New sensations, new journeys, different ways of doing things all stimulate the neurons to make new connections and thus keep our thinking and sensing faculties alive.

Memory Exercise 3: Learn Language

Learning new words or learning a new language provides enormous stimulation for the brain. There are several regions in both hemi-spheres of the brain involved with language. One area, called Wernick's area, in the posterior temporal lobe of the cerebral cortex of only one of the hemispheres (usually but not always the left), is asso-ciated with the "sound" of the language and is activated by trying to pronounce new words, particularly if they are of another language. Comprehension of language actually occurs in the prefrontal area, while the emotional component of language stimulates yet another area. Whenever you involve yourself in learning new words, playing word games, or learning a new language, you are activating all these areas of the brain.

Getting in Touch

Heart energy is expressed through the eyes and the touch of the hands. When we experience the heart as full and present, without fear, we are able to reach out through the eyes and hands to give and receive.

LINDA HARTLEY[1]

The skin, that boundary between inner and outer, self and not-self, is not only an exquisitely sensitive organ, it is also the largest organ of the body. It has a thin epidermis which provides us with protection and a thicker dermis below that. In addition to small capillaries which carry blood to it, it has minute and numerous nerve fibers that end in touch receptors. These receptors vary in size and shape and are designed to detect even the most subtle changes in our environment. Because we usually engage our awareness (buddhi) with the workings and projections of the ahamkara and the mind, we are not always aware of what we are touching or being touched by.

Touch Exercise 1: Engage your Attention

Take time out each day simply to engage your attention fully. During this time suspend judgments like "beautiful," "ordinary," "nice," "dull," etc., and simply become attentive.

I try to do this each day as dawn breaks, a time the Yogis call the brahmamahurta, the time of the Divine, by just stepping into my own back garden.

Here is how to use this technique:

- Instead of "thinking about" the scene, see all that there is to see, then close your eyes and smell all that there is to smell, hear all that there is to hear, become aware even of the taste on your tongue and feel the touch of the ground beneath your feet and the air against your skin (if you have a private garden and can do this naked, so much the better).

- That same evening take some time out again when you are indoors and all is quiet and allow your mind to recall all that you experienced during your morning attention burst. Write it down in a journal if you think that will help.

It does not matter that you may be viewing the same scene every day – as you grow more and more attentive you will see how many extraordinary changes there are to the scene as each day passes.

Touch Exercise 2: Use Your Sense of Touch

This is an extremely enjoyable exercise and almost everyone I have given it to says they have found it the most direct route to living from the heart that they have experienced.

- Choose an everyday task that you have done countless times, so much so that you can do it without thinking about it. (I chose washing the dishes as my first exercise; someone else chose making the journey from their car to their front door, finding the key and then opening it.)

- You are going to do the task just as you have always done it, but this time you are going to do it blindfold, using only your sense of touch to guide you.

Remember throughout the exercise that the hands are the instruments of the heart and that the sensations you are experiencing are being "felt" by the heart.

Touch Exercise 3: Sensitize Your Touch

This is an exercise used by many bodyworkers, for example massage therapists, to improve the "listening" ability of their hands when they explore the muscles of the body.

- Get a telephone book that has thin pages.

- Take a single strand of hair and place it under a page, then run your hand over the surface of the page and feel for the hair.

- Once you can easily detect the presence of the hair through one page, try it through two, and so on.

Because the hands are connected to the heart, as you sensitize the sense of touch in the hands you activate Anahata Chakra, enlivening Vayu – Wind – Tattva.

Touch Exercise 4: Develop Your Touch

Approach this next exercise with curiosity and in the spirit of inquiry!

Next time you are in the supermarket, buy two potted plants that you can grow on a windowsill indoors. Get two of the same species, state of health, and stage of growth, and take them home and give them both the water and care they need to thrive. Once they have settled into their new home – in about three weeks – you are going to see if you can train yourself to sense their vitality field, developing your sense of touch to a high degree.

- Place both plants where you can have easy access to them for the duration of the practice.

- Rub the palms of your hands together for a few seconds until they tingle, then blow on them, taking them to a heightened sensitivity.

- Allow your shoulders to relax, then move your hands wide apart with the palms facing each other.

- Slowly bring the hands towards each other until you feel a change. Some people feel as if the hands are suddenly pulling towards each other, others as if the hands are suddenly repulsing each other, yet others feel warmth. Whatever you feel is valid for you. Once you have felt a difference, you have been in touch with your own vitality field.

- Now try the same thing with each plant in turn. If your hands have lost sensitivity, rub and blow on them again. Hold them away from the plant and then slowly bring them towards the plant. Become aware of when you feel the vitality field of the plant by feeling a change.

- See if both plants feel the same. Is one vitality field stronger than the other, bigger than the other?

- Try placing one plant in less ideal conditions that the other, and practice the same exercise to see if the change in location has made a difference to the vitality field.

- During the next two weeks keep the plant in its unsuitable location and repeat the awareness exercise, noting any differences you may feel in both plants. Suspend judgment – just feel, and note down all that you feel. You are attempting to "feel" any distress before the plant shows visible signs of it.

- As soon as you are aware of any distress, move the plant back to its more suitable location.

Reconnecting to our Sensual Being

At the very moment when I live in the world, when I am given over to my plans, my occupations, my friends, my memories, I can close my eyes, lie down, listen to the blood pulsating in my ears, lose myself in some pleasure or pain, and shut myself up in this anonymous life... But precisely because my body can shut itself off from the world, it is also what opens me out upon the world and places me in a situation there.

MAURICE MERLEAU-PONTY[2]

We can land men and machines on the moon and yet we still fail to make a soft landing within the space of our own bodies. We can have "out of body" experiences and report contact with aliens and yet we still fail to make contact with our most basic physical needs and to be truly alive within the boundary of our own skin. In spite of and often because of these new sciences, we still close off to the body. We have simply added science to religious prohibition in denying the sacred as it is expressed in flesh and bone. And yet it is through the body that we live and age and enter into relation with this world.

Walking the road back to the body, engaging with its sensations and feelings without the mediation of religion or science and with a full realization of the spirit burning deep within its every cell, breath, and gesture, is a journey long overdue. It is a journey we must all make if we are to restore ourselves to a true sense of touch and be at peace with ourselves and our environment.

Our whole education still supports the view that thinking is better than being. It is not surprising, given this history, that most of us arrive in adulthood as what a friend called "heads on sticks." That is to say, we have successfully been taught to be alienated from our own feelings and to honor in ourselves only our so-called "rational processes." Feelings, including sexual feelings, are never rational – they are impulsive, often overwhelming, and playful things that call our attention when we least expect them. Too many people deny them any kind of response that honors them as a valid and sacred part of themselves.

Even if you are voluntarily or involuntarily celibate, awareness of sexuality is essential, as it is closely linked to the flow of vitality. If we suppress our sexuality, that vitality becomes distorted and blocked in many areas of the body. Whether you are engaging in sex or not, awareness is the sacred place between suppression and expression.

Family Mythologies

Give yourself time to consider the family mythologies you grew up with regarding sex, and how these have influenced your attitudes and sexual life.

As part of this exploration, write down in a journal how your past has influenced your feelings about sexuality now.

The Peripheral Nervous System

The peripheral nervous system – that part of the nervous system that exists outside the skull and spine – is itself so complex that divisions and sub-divisions are made of it for purposes of understanding it more fully. One of these sub-divisions is into the somatic and autonomic nervous systems:

⊚ The somatic nervous system conducts impulses from the brain to the skeletal muscles that allow us to make voluntary movements.

◎   The autonomic nervous system controls all those activities not under our voluntary control, like the rate of our heartbeat and breathing.

◎   The autonomic nervous system is again divided into two: the sympathetic and the parasympathetic nervous systems. Broadly speaking, the sympathetic nervous system stimulates us to be on the alert, while the parasympathetic nervous system calms us down. The sympathetic nervous system is all about dealing with the world, and the parasympathetic nervous system deals with internal "housekeeping" functions like maintaining the immune system.

In this ultra-fast world of bustle, most of us are working with over-activated sympathetic nervous systems and the functions of the parasympathetic nervous system are being deprived of vitality. To achieve balance, a state of sattva, we must pay as much attention to our internal environment as to our external. We must make time and space in our lives for such attention and that attention should take the form of silence, for it is in silence that our inner life is revealed.

One question that may be asked of this silence is: "Where am I going?"

Meditation: "Where Am I Going?"

This meditation can be done as a regular practice or when you find yourself in a difficult situation, particularly one where a decision has to be made. I also advise it if you are in conflict with someone, perhaps a friend or neighbor. Having some knowledge of where your current attitudes, feelings, and actions will take you clears the way for your spiritual journey right now.

•   Find a place and time that is going to be interruption-free for at least 20 minutes.

- Sit comfortably in a chair that allows your back, neck, and head to flow in a straight line; release your shoulders and allow the muscles at the back of your neck to lengthen; let your weight sink down into the chair beneath you.

- Take your awareness to your breath, feeling the movement in your abdomen, chest, and ribs as you breathe in and out.

- Feel the cool air entering your nose on the in-breath, flowing down your throat and warming as it enters your body, and then feel the warm breath flowing up through your throat and leaving through your nose.

- For a few moments let your awareness follow the out-breath to that brief stillpoint between breaths. Stay focused there and watch for the very first movement that will give rise to the next breath.

- Now bring to mind the current state of events in your life and all the attitudes, opinions, thoughts, and beliefs that you hold around these events.

- Simply hold the awareness in stillness to watch what the mind produces without making any judgments.

- In that stillness the most important features, people, and attitudes will emerge.

- Now project this into a future in which you will have changed no one else's mind about anything. The state of play is your state. Where do your current feelings, beliefs, and thoughts take you?

- Look at the image, the picture you are being given, and note carefully your internal responses to the landscape.

- Come back to your breath.

- Ask yourself in the truth of that stillness if there is an alternative road.

By awarding yourself time to maintain your memory and your sense of touch and stay deeply connected to who you are and where you are in relation with the world, you call on all the vitality of the Universe. Taking the time for these practices is time you have earned by living your life and being the person life called you to be.

The Fourth Wave

Chapter 9

Re-create Yourself

Some smart marketing man once said that if you tell a lie often enough it begins to take on the appearance of truth. One such lie is that our bodies are like machines. It all began when men began to manufacture machines, in particular the clock. In every way the clock is a contrast to the chaotic creativity of nature: in its mechanism there is order and precision. Life, on the other hand, tends to subordinate order to creativity.

No machine repairs, renews, or re-creates itself, but the living body is doing it all the time. Every year 98 per cent of the atoms in our bodies are replaced. It takes just six weeks for us to renew our outer covering of skin, eight weeks to renew our liver, and just five days to renew the stomach lining. This endless surge of building up and breaking down is one of the chief characteristics of life. No machine can do it – only living things have this alchemy.

Life came to planet Earth some 4,000 million years ago, taking the same stuff that makes stars and stardust, mixing a chemical here and a gas there, and forming itself into a single cell. Through a process of intimate alliances, mergers, and synthesis, it kept re-creating and transforming itself – and it continues to do so. Every time life seems doomed, it changes the plot and re-emerges. Its attachment to one particular form is never so total that it is not able to abandon it for another that seems more suited to its exuberance.

In the 1970s, two Chilean biologists, Francisco Varela (who has since died) and Humberto Maturana, came up with a remarkable theory of life that they labeled autopoiesis. Auto means "self" and poiein means "making." Autopoiesis is the theory that life is "self-making" or, to put it another way, life is involved in the constant and continuous re-creation of itself. By movement, by chemical exchange, by energy expenditure, life produces more life. It is engaged in a dance that produces the tender unfurling leaf of a fern and the hand holding the hammer banging the nail. It does not simply and endlessly reproduce more of the same, it diversifies and tries out new forms, new shapes.

Thought, however, styled and maintained by whatever culture shapes our identity, creates an image of ourselves that we grow up wholly committed to. And the hardest thing to change is that image. Despite the profound changes we witness around us every day, seeing our children grow and age, seeing the world change, seeing ourselves change, we hold onto that image and demand that it does not change. Any external force that demands the image be changed is met with the fiercest opposition we can muster.

Through the previous three waves we have been exploring that image. Now our self-examination has to rise to the challenge of continually transforming it. If we do not, if we maintain a defensive posture when called upon to examine what it is we think and believe we are, then we are truly committed to idol worship. Whenever we try to make this changing world conform to our image of non-change, we are idolaters. Then we buy into the fear of the younger generations which says that the changes that aging brings should not be experienced but treated like a disease that needs curing. Embracing these changes means accepting our changing role and affirming ourselves as the elders who teach our community about the adventures of aging. On the other hand, if we use aging as an excuse to rigidify, to cease changing, to cease re-creating ourselves, to cease producing more life, we lose the very essence of what life is all about.

The throat chakra, Vishuddha Chakra, houses the tattva of Space, the organizational capacity of creation to move from chaos to self-organization. Resisting that self-awareness means resisting also the impulse and movement of life, which continues transforming itself until it is fully self-aware. In that resistance we send Space Tattva into a tamasic state as the vitality streams from it to seek that point of creation, re-creation, and life-organizing-life elsewhere.

The degree of success we have at becoming wise seems to depend on our commitment to adapting to change. The flexibility of the body that we gain by remaining active should be mirrored by a commitment to keeping the inner instrument equally flexible. When we become fixed in certain emotional responses or ideas or belief systems, when we refuse to allow anything to enter, to touch us, we rigidify the inner instrument and it begins to lose its power for growth. When we conceive of aging as degeneration and attempt to claw back youth – an impossible task – we lose the possibility for growth that can take us into new areas of discovery and joy.

We have to become as flexible as Grandma Moses. When the American artist Ann May Moses's right hand became too swollen and painful with arthritis at the age of 70 to be able to continue with her beloved embroidery work, she switched to painting with her left hand. When her sight failed as she aged, she awakened her inner vision and painted remembered scenes from her childhood in happier times before the Great War. Her extraordinary career, that embraced not only art but also raising a family and farming, along with considerable marketing skills, continued till her death at the age of 101 in December 1961.

The wisest thing we can do as we age is to surrender our rigidities, grab on to the creative coat-tails of ever-changing life and flow with it.

Movement is Life

There is a story that Pythagoras, the Greek philosopher whom we call the father of mathematics, traveled to the Middle East to enter a school and further his education. But he was refused entry until he underwent a certain ritual fasting and cleansing technique. Annoyed, Pythagoras said he was not interested in rituals, only in knowledge, to which the school elders replied, "But we cannot give you knowledge until you have changed."

Changing ourselves is the basis of gaining knowledge and wisdom. Changing our direction if the road we are traveling is leading nowhere is the way of arriving at our destination. When we have uncovered the dream, whether it is Elise's desire to be an artist or Pythagoras's desire to be a physician, we must mark the way of getting there as clearly as the nerve impulses mark their route. Often that means adapting or letting go of those things which are no longer serving us, just as Joe had to let go of his anger.

Edna, Elise, Joe, Maureen – all of them had to allow themselves to be transformed rather than defending the position they found themselves in. That transformation occurs because we let go of the image long enough to allow the Self to become the guiding force of the ahamkara rather than the other way round.

Knowing something of the body, of its biology, gives us glimpses of the Self. Connective tissue that enfolds and penetrates every cell of the body reminds us of our interconnectedness. Muscles that contract to hold our dreams or our pain until it is safe to release them remind us that this creation is powered by a benign force. A heart that itself remains empty while it ceaselessly works to fill every other cell reminds us that one of the characteristics of this Self must be an almost incomprehensible kind of love. And the lightning-fast nervous system that calls us to connection and exploration reminds us that we are here because Life called us into being with a purpose that must be fulfilled.

The magical cell that continues to renew itself and in so doing renews the flow of life through us should remind us that this is an endless universe of infinite possibilities. Thus we see that the outer instrument, the body, is not divorced from the spirit, but is a particular expression of it. And yet that Self has a capacity that the body and personality do not: consciousness. Whatever self-awareness body, mind, and personality do possess is a reflection of the consciousness of that Self, the Inner Knower, Prajna, which creates continuity, wholeness, and homogeneity from all the diverse experiences of our lives.

The Pathless Land

Examination of the fragments does not bring about the comprehension of the totality.

SWAMI VENKATESANANDA[1]

However, identifying with this Self is the aspect of life's journey that most of us resist. We want to remain exactly what we are, surrender nothing of ourselves, just make a tweak here and a dent there, so that we can be happy.

When we have done great buckets of work on the outer and the inner instruments we expect life to flow smoothly from then on – no more sorrow, no more pain. But still they come. Having taken on the enormous task of realigning our physical bodies through changing our diet, our exercise routines, our entire lifestyle, and transforming the inner instrument through meditation, we become aware that both happiness and unhappiness still exist for us.

We might turn to building empires to stave off unhappiness. We use our enormous creativity to invent reasons for it: "It's his fault." We even create philosophies and belief systems: "A satanic force at work" or "Ultimately we all cause our own suffering." The empires crumble and leave only their rubble behind in the form of our pain, suffering, and isolation. All of the reasons, the "causes," for our unhappiness are what we have heard and accepted – they are fragments, not what we ourselves have experienced as Truth.

If you taste sugar, you immediately know sweet. But if someone comes along and tells you that in this encyclopedia or that scripture it says sweet tastes like this or like that, even though you may fully embrace the information or doctrine, commit it to memory and even die defending it, you do not know sweet, you have not experienced it. Knowing is something else entirely, and it requires that we bring all of ourselves now to focus on what knowing is.

Riding these waves into aging does not ensure that sorrow will avoid us or that we will have a protective shield against it. But now we are ready for the final transformation in which happiness and unhappiness take their proper place.

Aging is not for sissies.

ART LINKLETTER

We have to make this journey into aging with knowledge of the True Self within, not with a philosophy or belief system about it.

We have to know this Self that is the portal to the vast unfath-
omable Infinite Self and know too its relation to the rest of the
world. If we forget this Self, then the body becomes the cloak that
hides it – the cascades of chemical and neuronal signals that activate heart, muscle, and bone will mask it rather than reveal it. The
outer effort we make must correspond to an inner transformation.

The ahamkara may be translated as "the ego," but this transla-
tion is so familiar to us that we slide over it without truly grasping
its significance. The ahamkara takes on the roles that it needs to –
daughter, son, sister, mother, father, employee, employer, rich,
poor, happy, sad, optimistic, pessimistic – endless, endless labels
that it adopts in order to function in the world. The ahamkara
loves labels and identity tags because they define, and because it
can understand and work with them. Infinity, on the other hand, it
cannot comprehend, it can only be absorbed back into it.

Therein lies the resistance to this part of the journey. When we
say "I," we are referring only to the labels the ahamkara has adopted and chosen to define itself by. But when we say "I" and also
mean our infinite, eternal nature, we will have transformed our
awareness wholly. If this feels like giving "yourself" up, you have
understood the situation perfectly, because that is exactly what it is.
But in this surrender your ultimate purpose will have been fulfilled.

Remember the nerve signals that travel along nerve pathways
at unimaginable speed? These signals are able to negotiate synapses – gaps between nerve endings – without scrambling. In an
ingeniously magical moment, the signal changes from a largely
electrical one to a chemical one that negotiates the space of the
synapse, is picked up by the next nerve fiber and then continues on
its way once again converted into an electrical signal. It changes
constantly in order to reach its destination whole and intact.
nd then it surrenders itself. And as it ceases to be its purpose is

fulfilled: a breath is drawn, a hand reaches out, a heart beats. Potential is transformed into action.

In the same way we have to surrender in order to complete our transformation. Our renewal, our complete transformation, requires this kind of dynamic surrender of the ahamkara, the idea-of-I.

The Self that is consciousness remains consciousness regardless of the changes that we flow through. That Self is what we uncover as we align the body, the ahamkara, the mind and the awareness to its purpose. The ahamkara takes its original blueprint, its instruction to be, from the Self, just as the cell takes its instruction from the DNA. But then it takes on the shades and coloring of experience, becoming shaped by the mind that is taking in information from the world via the senses. The ahamkara then becomes the self that life constructs – it is the self that functions as an individual in a world formed by the experiences of being that individual.

When we engage in exercises that uncover past dreams and past pain, it is the ahamkara that we are uncovering and transforming. It is the "I" that has broken itself off from infinity and fragmented itself by being committed to this time and this place. The first steps on the journey towards that Self must be to align the rest of the being, including the ahamkara, with it and its purpose. That, first of all, means being courageous enough to question the position of the ahamkara in all of its relationships.

"Isvara pranidhanad va," "Come into perfect alignment with That," declared the great codifier of Yoga, the sage Patanjali, 2,500 years ago. Isvara means "That One which Is" – the unborn Self. Patanjali tells us that the path to freedom and enlightenment, in which we no longer mistake ourselves for the limited and know ourselves to be limitless, is by aligning what we now believe ourselves to be with That. Then complete transformation becomes possible.

> ... and you shall know the truth
> and the truth shall set you free.

THE GOSPEL OF JOHN 8:32

This is the most powerful act of the body/mind complex, and it is almost impossible to accomplish in youth, when life seeks to be renewed through us by procreation. In youth our creativity revolves around the perpetuation of our species – and we heroically bring much more to it than simple reproduction. The way we have organized ourselves socially in order to reproduce has made us one of the most successful species on Earth and is a testament to our ingenuity. But as we age life gives us back to our soul's purpose and we can look to the re-creation of ourselves.

This requires an enormous leap of faith, the kind of leap the electrical nerve signal makes on leaving the end of the nerve fiber. As it makes that leap it might not know what it will become – but it knows it is born to make that leap. Our faith should be as sure.

The spiritual journey is a process of aligning with the True Self. The ahamkara, the I-maker or the idea-of-I, is extremely dense and until now we have been working on exposing its many layers to our own consciousness. The changes that Edna, Elise, Joe, and Maureen were making allowed each ahamkara to fulfill itself. They had been living lives in which the awareness (buddhi) was totally absorbed by one facet of the ahamkara. In order to release the awareness they had to allow other facets of the ahamkara to unfold and be expressed. This fulfillment of the ahamkara in the world is the first part of the spiritual journey, mirrored in the body as the transformation that the nerve signal makes to leap a synapse before continuing its journey.

The next part of the journey is to expand the attention of the awareness from the ahamakara to that other part of the self – the eternal Self within. From this expanded awareness the position of the ahamkara is again made conscious.

Finally, for complete transformation, the ahamkara must surrender itself to the True Self – like the nerve signal surrendering itself at the end of the nerve fiber to become the action.

Completing this transformation requires that you

Re-create Yourself

constantly in order to uncover all that you are, traveling always from potential to action.

As we come to this wave we are far out on the ocean and growing in strength by navigating these waters. Now it is time, even while we do not let the shore slip from our awareness, to begin to understand that we are no longer tied to it – we have set ourselves free for the process of transformation to become even more focused. Youth might have the capacity for physical growth, but it is old age that holds the promise of a total makeover!

By choosing to work against the habits of a lifetime we choose a holistic life. The word "holistic" comes from the Greek holos, which means "whole." It implies a reality of complementary and integrated parts. As we ride this wave we begin to bring these parts into an integrated whole which encompasses the True Self as it mirrors the Infinite.

The Time is Right

Nuncle, thou shouldst have grown wise ere thou grewest grey.

SHAKESPEARE, *KING LEAR*

There are both ancient and contemporary perspectives on spirituality which envision aging as the culmination of a process of change and spiritual evolution. A dear friend and brother in spirit, Diederick Reineke, having successfully taken to the ocean of aging, shared with me a system that comes from anthroposophy, founded by Rudolph Steiner. Diederick explained the system in this way:

> Between our 21st and 42nd years we are in a kind of probation period where we are given those trials that are meant to strengthen us. It is a time ruled by the Sun, when we make the struggle to be who we are meant to be. That is why these are often the years of our deepest despair as we waver between confidence and doubt, often unsure whether we have it in us to manifest what we have to bring forth.
>
> From 42 to 49 are the years of Mars, the time when you manifest and establish all that you have been working towards, provided that you have made yourself an efficient enough vehicle for your will. As our 49th year ends, according to this philosophy, all unfolding and repercussions of past actions, all karma that has shadowed us and informed our lives, ends. From this year forward we can choose our own direction, free from karmic influences.
>
> In the years between 49 and 56 we are governed by benign Jupiter, which brings us tolerance and the ability to reflect on our lives.
>
> Then comes the time from 56 to 63, when righteousness becomes the imperative. Ruled by distant Saturn, we are called into spiritual uprightness. All this growth occurs in order that by the time we are 63 we enter the years of being the sage, under the rule of the Universe, the "infinite horizon."

Diederick is now battling cancer, one of the many demons that rears its head more frequently as we age, reminding us that we must ask the urgent questions of ourselves. He lets himself be guided by the principles of these stages. He is seeking out that which he needs now to seek – knowledge of the Self. He is committing the image he has of himself to the fire of self-inquiry. He is still a husband and a father, still a teacher, still a brother, but the emphasis has been entirely transformed. He uses the menace of his brain tumor to remind himself of the ultimate journey, the journey the ahamkara must make to merge with the Self. As he makes this journey, his identity is no longer bound to the ahamkara, and in his presence the light of that Self can be glimpsed by all of us even as he is being transformed by it.

As we age, the energy cluster or chakra at the crown of the head which called us into standing upright to view a greater horizon in our evolution, and which plays out this same call in each child's life as it learns to stand up, now calls us into spiritual uprightness. Diederick is heeding the warning of King Lear's jester, becoming wise as he becomes gray. Like him we have to approach the Self which is at the heart of all.

The question here becomes: "Who am I?"

We are on the ocean and what those still confined to the shore cannot see is that now the ocean must become a fire. Now the ahamkara must be the fuel for the fire. Like the nerve signal it must surrender itself in order to be fulfilled. The aware Self will entirely transform the ahamkara into its own image when we make that surrender – so that we finally realize the truth of the contract that we are all made in the image of God.

The fire is vichara, direct observation. Into its blaze we place everything. In this direct observation we begin the process of withdrawing the awareness, the buddhi, from its flow outwards to the body, the personality and the many relations they have made with the world. We do not lose touch with these, but we do not lose ourselves in them either. In this process we move the vitality into a balanced – sattvic – state so that it is ready for that leap from potential into action. Only in that state of perfect poise and balance can we become wholly present to that Presence within, re-creating ourselves in the image of That.

The One eternal amidst the momentary,
The supremely conscious among the conscious,
The One who is their desires
And the fulfillment of their desires –
The wise are they who see That.
They have peace, no others.

THE BRHADARANYAKA UPANISHAD[2]

In *The Brhadaranyaka Upanishad* the sage Yajnavalkya is preparing to retire into the forest in order to spend his last years in solitude, so he calls his two wives to him and informs them that he is taking to the final stage of life and that he has left them both all his wealth, equally apportioned. They will be rich and able to live out their remaining years in comfort. One wife, Katyayani, is delighted and gets ready to go off with the goods. But the other wife, Maitreyi, hesitates and asks him, "Will this wealth that you are offering me also give me knowledge of immortality?" "No," the sage replies, "Wealth is not meant to do that but it will give you comfort and some power in the world." "That's not good enough," Maitreyi replies. "Give all the wealth to Katyayani if you like, if it doesn't confer the ultimate knowledge on me, I am not interested." Maitreyi thus instantly transforms herself from a wife into a spiritual student, and Yajnavalkya is transformed from a husband into a spiritual teacher. Both are transforming the ahamkara to the call of the inner purpose.

You can carry on worshipping the image you have of yourself, the role that you are now playing. But this will leave you gray, not wise. You may have transformed your appearance, but not your idea-of-I with all its fears, all its hang-ups, all its joys, all its pain. If you have navigated the waters this far and now stop, you will have seen the waves but you will not know that you are the ocean.

By taking to the wave of re-creating ourselves we challenge the foundations of what we believe ourselves to be and we question the postures the ahamkara adopts, keeping it always moving towards balance – sattva – as we observe it with extraordinary focus and attention. That is vichara.

Direct Observation

Nothing is loved for its own sake –
Everything is loved for the sake of the Self.

SAGE SAJNAVALKYA, *THE BRHADRYANYAKA UPANISHAD* 2:4:5[3]

The I-maker has come to believe that it is the subject, and that whatever it loves or is attracted to is an object outside itself. Not so, says Yajnavalkya to his disciple and former wife. It is drawn to the "object" because the same Self that exists in us exists also in the object – it is universal. It does not matter if the object is another person, the beloved, or something inanimate.

Mary believes she is in love with Mike because he's kind and humorous and gorgeous. Not so, says the sage. That is what the ahamkara sees, but the force behind it is the Self that is being drawn to itself, there is no lover and there is no beloved, there is just One.

... the primary emphasis is now on undivided wholeness, in which the observing instrument is not separated from what is being observed.

DAVID BOHM AND DAVID PLEAT, PHYSICISTS[4]

What, after all, is the subject and what is the object? I, Swami Ambikananda, am the subject, but the "object" of my love and affection is also a subject, not merely an object with some relation to me.

So the question becomes: "What is the subject? What is the object? Who am I?"

As quantum physics is discovering in its discussion of observer and observed, somewhere between these two lies Truth. To uncover it, to move towards that moment when the ahamkara is totally absorbed and therefore completely and finally transformed, we ride this wave of re-creating ourselves. This re-creation is not simply changing the body and mind but final and complete transformation in which the "I" of the ahamkara is surrendered to fulfil the purpose of the universal Self.

This is only possible when we allow vichara to become as necessary as breathing, when we let the awareness move to follow every movement – of body, of thought, of emotion.

Vichara is a dynamic and vital process. It is not something which is a dull routine or habit. The very essence of vichara is vitality: it must be alive.

SWAMI VENKATESANANDA[5]

To bring about this transformation the ancient rishis used to retreat into the forest. But we live in a new time, making the journey into aging and embracing the call of the Self amidst the abundance and confidence of youth. Surrounded by unyielding asphalt and concrete, we have to find the courage to simplify our lives and sharpen our focus to make the same journey as the ancients, struggling past the I-maker to our final transformation, towards wholeness. This is the wave that calls on us to make the ultimate paradigm shift, the internal movement in our lives that does not reject life but focuses our awareness in another direction, inward towards that zero point, the bindu, where creation and re-creation begin.

In this re-creation of ourselves the observer and the observed merge into pure awareness. The primal wound that fractured these two apart is healed, and as it is healed it becomes a point of healing for everyone. No longer isolated, we now "know" through direct experience our oneness with all – we are made sacred and the vitality that flows through the universe finds in us a river through which it can sustain the flow of life.

> Unmoving, the Self moves,
> Moving, it remains ever still.
> How is it known –
> That which is beyond all joy and sorrow
> And yet is embodied in both the joyful and the sorrowing?

> One who meditates on that Self
> Which is formless in the midst of all forms,
> Eternal in the midst of the momentary,
> Which is everywhere at once ...
> Such a one will know that Self
> And finally cease grieving.

THE KATHA UPANISHAD 2:21 AND 22[6]

Chapter 10

Riding the Wave
of Re-creating Yourself

Consciousness is universal and indivisible: it is one and it alone
is diverse.

SWAMI VENKATESANANDA[1]

We have so long been educated that existence is a hierarchy with
God and angels at the top and human beings somewhere near the
bottom but above animals and insects and maybe rocks and whole
planets that it takes an enormous shift in our thinking to begin to
see Divinity, spirit, matter, and consciousness all as one continuous
state of being.

Strangely, it is science rather than religion that is giving us new
heart in this spiritual search for ourselves as a part of a spiritual
whole. Science is now admitting that there is much more to reality
than the common-sense "objective" universe we are accustomed
to seeing.

We used to think that atoms were exactly like the sun with
planets orbiting around its gravitational field, only in the case of the
atom it was electrons circling round the nucleus. Everything was
fixed and that fixedness gave rise to the world that we see. This
view made nature predictable, just as the orbits of the planets are

predictable. Then came the astonishing and awe-inspiring discoveries from early last century that revealed that solid matter was not so solid after all – and predictability gave way to uncertainty.

The ahamkara always rebels against uncertainty. It can only function in the field of what the ancients called maya. The word maya comes from the Sanskrit root ma, meaning "to measure." The ahamkara works within a field that can be measured and in which predictable measurements can be made. Once, through meditation, you have become accustomed to the dialogue your mind is constantly engaged in, you will notice how much of that engagement involves going over events of the past and projecting possible outcomes and actions for the future – measuring and predicting.

Quantum physics, the new science which acknowledges a reality where uncertainty and unpredictability also operate, is not the way the ahamkara experiences the world. The ahamkara experiences the pavement beneath our feet and the money in our wallets and assigns them a value in relation to itself. The new physics says that that is not the only reality but simply one aspect of it and the other is that the dancing, moving atomic particles exist in a dual state of both particle and wave. The particle bit is easy for us to understand – it is a concentrated lump (however small) of something solid. The wave nature is a bit more challenging. It is not a wave like a sound wave but more like a crime wave. When we speak of a crime wave hitting a particular town, we are simply saying that crime in that town has increased to the extent that we are more likely to encounter a crime there than in another town. It's exactly the same with the wave nature of so-called solid matter: if you want to find a solid particle, you look in the place where the wave is strongest. But the truth is no one can accurately predict where the particle will appear, only where it is likely to do so. You could stand around on the street corner of the town hit by the crime wave for weeks and nothing may happen to you. On the other hand you may get mugged in the town where there is no crime wave. That is how solid matter is – more likely to appear in one place, but it is just as likely to appear somewhere else.

In it all is the element of unpredictability and interaction between observer and that which is being observed. The reality that the ahamkara assigns to pavement or money is simply that – the reality it has chosen as an observer out of many possible realities. But move beyond it and you enter the world where the distinction between observer and the observed become blurred, and all things become possible. Meditation, expanding the consciousness, the buddhi, allows us to move our awareness to that part of the field of being where creativity is directed.

> Quantum physics undermines materialism because it reveals that matter has far less "substance" than we might believe ... In this "overthrow of matter," writes Gilder, "the powers of mind are everywhere ascendant over the brute force of things."

DAVIES AND GRIBBIN[2]

Quantum physics developed and expanded as we who are now reaching middle and old age were growing up, and it informs us that change is the order of the universe. Nothing is pre-determined and everything is open to exciting possibilities. What hope! The gift of creation and re-creation remains with us.

We need this information as we enter the journey of aging. Everyone around us, from the youth-obsessed media to the pharmaceutical industry, is going to be telling us, predicting for us, what aging will mean. We need to be able to look at this new science and know that it is within our own scope to define what our aging will mean for each of us.

Everything is made up of dancing atoms and yet I feel the pavement beneath my feet and the solidity of the money in my wallet. Science is saying that perhaps these things are there because you expect them to be there. One scientist put it beautifully (and tantalizingly) when he said that the wave-like and ghostly world of the atom only transforms into concrete reality when an observation is made – it only comes into being when you look at it, as if it knows that you are looking and what it is you expect to see. The exact nature of reality – my reality – requires my participation as an observer. It is not that the pavement and the banknotes are unreal, it is that my particular view of them and my absolute commitment to a particular "reality" engage with them – they are not what they are without my participation.

John Wheeler, a physicist from the University of Texas, makes it even more astonishing. Conscious observation, he says, is partially responsible even for past events, maybe even events that occurred before we were alive! Thus he presents the universe as "a self-observing system."

What we are in reality we do not yet know. Discovering the reality behind the appearance is the spiritual quest. The cells that make up our body are themselves made up of billions of atoms – as subject to these laws as the atoms of the pavement beneath my feet and the money in my wallet. This makes change, re-creation, transformation possible at any time.

As we age, if we allow even our views on the nature of reality to be challenged, we open up to the possibility of re-creating ourselves. When we know and honor this truth, we are aging wisely. We become shamans, living at the level of creativity and never offending the flow of life.

Shaking the Image of Who I Am

The more often a thought is imprinted in the mind, the more we accept it as truth and it becomes who we are. The 70-thousand-odd thoughts that we think each day are sadly made up of the same content day after day. For example, people who suffer from depression are often in the habit of thinking depressed thoughts.

Become attentive to unguarded thoughts in the same way that you became aware of anger. Commit yourself to writing not less than one page and not more than five pages every day of stream of consciousness-type "stuff." Then read what you have written. If you discover that your background dialogue is one of negativity, filled with what is not right with your life, what you have not received, how hopeless you are, you know that you have to change.

My teacher Swami Venkatesananda taught me this method of keeping a journal: I wrote in black ink on the right-hand page of the notebook, always leaving the left-hand page blank. When I (and he) read it, I was amazed at the stream of hopelessness that flowed from me at that time. He then asked me to choose a sentence I had written in black on the right-hand side of the page and rewrite it from a different point of view in red on the left-hand side. For example, when I didn't get up for meditation for a few mornings I had written in black ink about how lazy and no good I was and how I was sure to fail at Yoga as I had failed at everything else in my life. So I wrote in red ink on the opposite side that I had not got out of bed but had let my body and mind rest, and that when they had rested fully the impulse to meditate would surely reassert itself. When I wrote that I was just about the worst mother in the world and had no idea how my children would get to adulthood with me as a mother, he told me to write down in red that mothering was a tough job to hold down and what helped was knowing that my children's future was in the hands of life and their own spirit, not just mine.

The most important thing about your journal is that it should be is a safe place to keep a record of your own background dialogue and what your mind is producing. You are being your own confidant and guide through its pages.

It was by keeping a journal that I grew in awareness and understanding of the chakras. As we have seen, each chakra – Earth, Water, Fire, Air, and Space – imparts particular characteristics to the vitality flowing through it. For example, Muladhara Chakra transforms vitality to take on the characteristics of earth – solidity, support, and equanimity. If this chakra is balanced – in a sattvic state – then these properties will be balanced in us also. But if it becomes rajasic (overactive) or tamasic (inert), then this will also be reflected in body and personality. A tamasic Muladhara Chakra will not be producing enough earth-type energy to support our body mass and this may result in us losing physical mass, losing balance, etc. But it will also express itself in our moods, thoughts, and feelings. Perhaps we will have feelings of being unsupported by people around us, or our equanimity may give way to excessive worrying. On the other hand, a rajasic Muladhara Chakra may produce a sudden increase in mass as our consumption suddenly exceeds our needs; or we may begin to manipulate others and use the "pure" qualities of earth, like being supportive, simply to get things going our own way.

When my journal displayed signs of excessive worrying about very small things or signs of feeling sorry for myself, I could see how they reflected an imbalance in the chakras. For example, when I was confined to bed after some serious surgeries, Muladhara Chakra became tamasic (bed rest immediately disturbs Earth Tattva, which relies on the movement of bone and muscle to keep drawing on vitality). This was reflected in some serious worrying and whining in my journal and the love and support I was getting from the people around me never seemed to be enough – always a sure sign that Earth Tattva is out of balance.

When the chakras are in balance we just don't notice their existence, nor do we need to. But when they become imbalanced we can see what has gone wrong, and by working to change our thinking patterns we can actually alter the vitality flow through the chakras. Time and again the Yoga texts attest to the fact that the vitality follows the mind.

By keeping the ahamkara in a sattvic state we are aligning it with the purposes of the Self, enabling it to draw closer to surrender.

Use this chart to map the flow of vitality through the chakras, while observing the thought processes described through your journal.

Earth

Tamasic: Feeling unsupported; excessive worrying; anxiety; being insidiously manipulative; reminiscing about the "good old times;" excessive worrying about what others will think; loss of sense of smell.

Sattvic: Being considerate of self and others.

Rajasic: Being overly sympathetic; inappropriately taking on others' problems; being overly fearful of possible conflict; highly reactive sense of smell.

Water

Tamasic: Being very fearful about everything (particularly the future); loss of creative abilities and imagination; being withdrawn; loss of memory; excessive dreaming (mostly nightmares); procrastination; irritability; loss of sense of taste.

Sattvic: Strength of purpose; courage of convictions.

Rajasic: Seeing no obstacles to purpose; excessive daydreaming; beginning to blur lines between reality and imagination; making plans but being unable to put them into action.

Fire

Tamasic: Feeling stressed; loss of energy; loss of inner vision; loss of joy; pessimistic; easily angered; easily shocked; fearful of intimacy.

Sattvic: Clear vision of purpose.

Rajasic: Being excited about everything; impulsive; contemptuous of others; inner vision blocked, not being able to really see the way ahead but forging ahead anyway.

Air

Tamasic: Excessive self-involvement; taking no account of others' needs or plans; inability to go forward or to get out of situations not providing growth; tearful; aggressive; demanding; lack of introspection.

Sattvic: Assertion and leadership (without anger or aggression).

Rajasic: Anger and loss of temper; assertion of will over others; domineering; easily moved to tears; not feeling emotionally connected or "touched;" extremely aggressive; perceiving innocent remarks or actions as an attack.

Space

Tamasic: Feeling a sense of loss and/or isolation; inability to open up to others even if wanting to; losing touch with inner guiding voice; being obsessive about tidiness or cleanliness or order.

Sattvic: Open and appropriate control, letting go what is not needed.

Rajasic: Extreme sense of grief; keeping a tight lid on all emotions; loss of sense of control; feelings of powerlessness; loss of a sense of intimacy with others.

When you find tamasic or rajasic expressions of the tattvas entering your journal, find ways of introducing the sattvic pattern. Remind yourself of your direction and purpose by keeping images of yourself in the sattvic state of that tattva in mind throughout the day or week.

Keeping a journal in this way also allows you to see clearly that the ahamkara, with its likes and dislikes, positivity and negativity, is simply a construct. We committed to its patterns in a state of unconsciousness and now, as we become conscious, as we see it as it is, we withdraw our commitment from the limiting forces of both positivity and negativity to live and act in the sacred space between these opposite polarities.

Who Am I?

Direct Observation

Allow a quiet time of at least half an hour for meditation each day and include this exercise in some of your meditations.

- Sit on a chair or on the floor in a posture in which you are comfortable with your back, neck, and head flowing in a straight line.

- Observe the flow of breath as in the previous exercise.

- Now one by one begin to bring to mind the labels you have identified with up to now.

- Choose just one of those tags, for example your gender identity tag.

- Bring it into sharp focus and remain as aware as possible without letting the awareness slide into the mind's tendency to begin making judgments and labeling things as "good" or "bad," "right" or "wrong."

• Allow everything associated with that tag to come into view. For example, if you have chosen the gender tag, see what is attached to that role. You may argue that gender is not a role but a real biological fact. Absolutely true. I am a woman and there is no disputing that biological fact. But what it means to be a woman in my society and time is a construct of the I-makers that I grew up with or that I have embraced in my adulthood. For example, when I was studying Chinese medicine, a shiatsu teacher that I went to who was committed to Yin and Yang as gender polarities (Yin being "feminine" and Yang being "masculine") said I was denying my feminine nature by being forceful in my views. He had a definite idea of what a female should be, of what identity tags a woman should have, passivity being one of them. So society will have tagged you whether you are male or female, through the ahamkara that gathers roles and identities to itself as blotting paper absorbs water. Simply be aware of its roles, insofar as you can at this one sitting.

• Now if all these tags that go with being male or female are removed, what is there? What is the reality that emerges? What is?

Write down your observations in your journal and try a new identity role each time. You are working towards finding out the reality of who you are, rather than merely reacting.

Be careful here that you do not allow your mind to project an ideal of what you would like to be. That simply creates conflict. Let your attention stay with what is.

By adopting this meditation technique a patient was able to pull herself out of a long-standing dispute with her son and daughter-in-law that threatened the relationship with her grandchildren. When she had all her labels, prominent among them was "mother." When she examined it without being judgmental or defensive, she saw clearly that there was a load of "stuff" clinging to it that she had inherited from her own mother, things like "Mother should always be obeyed," "Mother is right," "Mother should be thought of before anyone else." She came out of the meditation realizing that she was presenting herself to her children in an unconscious way – that she had simply constructed the mother identity from the blueprint she had observed in her own mother. This awareness itself began to change her and her relationships, without her deciding that there was an ideal that she had to conform to.

Another exercise for experiencing the ahamkara and becoming more focused on our spiritual selves than its constructs is examining the identity tags we place on ourselves.

Discovering the Self beyond the Labels

Find a quiet time during which you can devote a full hour without interruptions to the following task:

- In your journal write down a list all your identity tags, everything that the ahamkara thinks that it is – male/female, daughter/son (even if your parents are no longer alive you are still their child), father/mother, friend, teacher, actress, secretary, shop assistant, CEO, dog owner, house owner, spiritual being, sister/brother, lover, Christian, Muslim, Buddhist, Hindu, etc. Just keep writing and writing until you have exhausted every label or identity tag you can think of.

- Set the journal aside for two weeks and then when things are quiet take it out and read through your labels. Are there any that need to be added – angry person, frightened person, disappointed person? Again, keep writing until you have exhausted all the labels that come to mind.

- When no more labels come to mind, sit quietly in that void and allow yourself to experience Reality beyond the ahamkara.

- Repeat this exercise regularly and be aware of the enormous change that is brought by this kind of observation.

> ... truly breath is the life of all beings,
> The Life of all life.
>
> *THE TAITTIRIYA UPANISHAD*[5]

Breath has a special place in our spiritual quest – among all cultures it is considered to be that which stands between matter and spirit and belongs to both worlds. We can use it to find the Oneness of these two states of being.

Once you have completed the above exercise you could go straight into this next meditation exercise:

The Breath inside the Breath

- Sit on a chair or on the floor in a posture in which you are comfortable, with your back, neck, and head flowing in a straight line.

- Allow your attention to flow towards the movement of breathing, feeling your abdomen expanding, bellowing out as you breathe in, and then contracting as you breathe out. Feel the slight movement of your chest lifting as you breathe in and then sinking as you breathe out. Feel your ribs lifting up and away from your hips and expanding as you breathe in and then contracting and sinking as you breathe out.

- Absorb your attention further and feel the sensations of breathing: the cool air entering your nose, hitting the back of your throat and warming as it enters your body and then the warm air rising up through your throat and leaving through your nose.

- Now let your attention follow the out-breath ... Stay with the out-breath. Watch it intently and stay with it as it ends. Stay with it during the stillpoint between breaths. Watch intently for the very first movement that gives rise to the next breath.

- Do not let the ahamkara intervene to take the next breath. Let that breath simply happen to you.

- Wait and watch to discover, to uncover, that which is breathing you.

Allowing the awareness to unmask the ahamkara and become aware of the Self is a total denial of the false identities our civilization, our culture, has put together over millennia. It is a denial of all the ugliness, corruption, brutality, and violence that we have perpetrated in our society. We see in this awareness that these things did not appear there by themselves – they exist outside ourselves because they exist within each one of us. They are what we expect to see outside ourselves because they exist within us.

We can begin to create a new state of being – the state of being that aging has called on us to create right now for our world. Such awareness is the surrender of the ahamkara to the Self. Once we deny the ahamkara with all its identities, the Self is, and its intelligence and grace act in our lives.

The Fifth Wave

Chapter 11

Turn and Face
the Other Way

See this world for what it is:
An illusion – no more substantial
Than a ring of fire
Traced by a burning torch in the dark;
An illusion coloured by the gunas
And shaped as form.
In Reality it is the One Pure Consciousness
Which appears as the many.

THE UDDHAVA GITA 8:34[1]

I sat at June's hospital bed watching the breathing pattern that often comes to the dying: her abdomen forcing air out and dragging it in increasing and decreasing bursts, in a process similar to what the ancient Yogis called bhastrika; in medicine it is called Cheyne-Stokes breathing. I have witnessed it many times in the dying and it usually signals that the end is drawing near – the *prana* using the dramatic movement in the muscles of the abdomen to complete its flow out of the body. Just a couple of hours earlier June and I had shared our last joke, and then she had closed her eyes and I could do nothing but be present and watch as the merry, intelligent, and affectionate manifestation that was my friend began to withdraw itself. Sometime in the early hours of the morning, in the time that belongs to fire and transformation, she breathed out and did not breathe in again.

For just a few seconds, as her presence no longer filled her body, I felt June all around me, in me, as if she was giving me a final and sweet gift: allowing me to feel her transition from a local event – the body – to a non-local, universal one.

Once we have learned to surrender the image of ourselves that we have nursed all through our adulthood, we are confronted by what seems to be the ultimate surrender – death.

Death dogs our path all through our lives and no matter how lively our step it is always just one pace behind for absolutely everybody. The language we use for it, rather than using the word itself, varies depending on our feelings at the time from "the final resting-place" to "the Grim Reaper." Pictorially, we usually represent it as a male figure in a dark hooded cloak with a scythe coming to cut us down. To my knowledge the only person who ever referred to death as female was the gentle St Francis of Assisi, who called death "our sister." And truly death is like a faithful sister who keeps us company every moment of our lives, reminding us not to forget our true nature, because that is what we will return to.

Whatever our feelings about death, one day it is suddenly in front of us. It is the ultimate moment of change that will come upon us all, regardless of social position, looks, abilities, wealth, or health. Sister Death is the great leveler and no one can peek beyond her veil.

"Tell me about life after death," requested the disciple.
"I cannot tell you that, I can only tell you that you must practice clear mind and peaceful heart," replied the Master.

"Well, aren't you supposed to be a Zen Master?" retorted the disciple.

"Yes," answered the Master, "but I am not a dead one."

ZEN STORY[2]

On the one hand we sense the eternal within ourselves, the forever 25-year-old, the Self, but on the other hand it looks out at this world through a body that is momentary. It seems it was not always so. At the very origins of life on this planet only accidents, some external cause, killed a living cell. Then at some point in evolution the humble but quite extraordinary cell, which can reproduce itself over and over, built death into its nature, and the truth is that we cannot be who and what we are without its orderly process.

At a certain stage in its life the cell produces the enzyme that it needs to destroy itself and it begins the process of dying. The enzyme initiates and oversees the cell's demise, packaging it up for use by adjacent cells and leaving its remains in a condition to be devoured by immune cells.

If a single cell fails to live by these rules and begins to multiply, it is a "rogue" that turns into a tumor – cancerous or non-cancerous – and threatens the entire organism. Our cells are dying all the time in order that we may live. But one day the process becomes global throughout the body and we die.

Soul to Cell

Prajna is seated within the heart ...

That state of deep sleep in which there is no dream,
In which the sleeper neither desires any object nor rejects it,

That is the third part and Prajna is active there.
This is the integrated bliss state
Which projects itself out to become body, mind and vitality.

THE MANDUKYA UPANISHAD 5[3]

The human body is made up of trillions of cells – about 200 varieties of them. Branching nerve cells, chubby round fat cells, strange cube-like cells of kidney tubules, long threadlike cells of muscles – on and on they go, each cell taking on a shape that suits its function. At the center of each cell is the nucleus, the center of being that tells the cell what it is and what it must be. Within the nucleus is the precious DNA, the genetic code that carries the entire life instruction for the cell. When an entire body, or even a cell of that body (like a sperm or an ovum), creates another similar being with distinct changes that come about due to a new genetic combination – a few mutations, maybe a developmental variation – that is creation, that is life. And in this the life of the cell is a perfect metaphor for the life of the Self that flows from the heart.

When we expand our attention to encompass that Self we begin to live a full life in which everything is transformed and limitations like birth and death take on an entirely different dimension. In this awareness we stand the most chance of changing the world, of healing the divisions and overcoming the obstacles that now stand before all of us – the folly of the way we have been living because we believed we were separate from one another.

How Far Can We Go?

Whither do the half-months and months go?
Whither the seasons with the year?

Whither the fruits of the seasons?
Speak to me of that ...

ATHARVA VEDA X.7.5

How far can we go? We can make our bodies grow stronger and our minds clearer, keep our hearts open and continually re-create ourselves, but none of these will stave off death. Amazingly, we find that even if medicine, with a wave of its magic pharmaceutical wand, were to suddenly wipe out cardiovascular disease, cancer, and even Alzheimer's, the average lifespan would only go up by another decade or so. Life, it seems, puts an end to each individual expression of itself.

"What is the cause of death?" a voice cried out from the crowd. The Enlightened One looked out with eyes of unending compassion and then he spoke.
"Birth," he replied.

STORY OF THE BUDDHA TOLD BY SWAMI VENKATESANANDA

We all die of something, and as we get older we are more likely to die than when we are young. In the United States and Europe, the death rate among children between birth and 12 years of age is very low, less than 1 in 1,000. By the time we reach our thirties it has gone up to just over 1 in 1,000, and by the time we are in our forties it has gone up to over 5 in 1,000. Then there are some big leaps: by the time we are in our sixties it is nearly 50 in 1,000, and in our seventies just over 80 in 1,000. The curve rises sharply as we age. "No man is free who fears death," said the Rev. Dr Martin Luther King, Jr. But we cannot bear the thought of our own death, our own "not being," and so we cover up the question with belief systems and philosophies. Rather than contemplating our own mortality and using it to transform our lives, we pursue physical immortality, as if matter and space are the only things that can possibly hold our consciousness.

"The Highly Gifted Son of Heaven," the Chinese Emperor Qin Shihuang, who built the Great Wall of China, founded its envied silk industry, and was finally buried somewhere near his vast terra-cotta army, was said to have spent many fortunes searching for the elixir of youth. It is now thought by some toxicologists that he probably died of heavy metal poisoning from the very potions that were meant to prolong his life! We might smile at such folly, but then we pick up a newspaper and it reads: "Anti-aging Breakthrough: Scientist Close to Longevity Pill" and we think, "Whoopee!" – until we read it. Somewhere in a remote laboratory some scientist has managed, over many years, to access the DNA of an earthworm and enhance its genetic structure to resist the wear and tear of life. How exactly this will translate for humans is a leap the news ignores. You do a bit of digging and you discover that it's a great idea, but they have absolutely no mechanism for delivering the miracle breakthrough to our 70-odd trillion cells. In fact, if they were able to deliver it to just one human cell that would be a real breakthrough.

Throughout history there have been many Highly Gifted Sons (and Daughters) of Heaven pursuing the prospect of physical immortality that could be just around the corner. But until they have rounded that corner – and they may, for our species is nothing if not inventive – we still have death on our doorstep.

How each of us deals with the thought of death will depend on the perspective we choose to adopt. If we adopt the perspective of science, then death is a problem to be solved. However, if we look at it from a spiritual perspective, it is a mystery to be uncovered. Each stage of life presents us with new mysteries and coming to terms with these mysteries is essential to successful aging. When we are children the mystery is adulthood; when we are teenagers the mystery is falling in love; when we are adults the mystery is the child being born; when we grow old the mystery is death.

A Question of Focus

As we age and begin to think of our own death, it is not immortality that we must seek but that in ourselves which is immortal.

We have been making ourselves familiar with a model of the tattvas bound together: space (Akasha Tattva), movement (Vayu Tattva, which includes the movement of linear time), and matter (Earth, Water, and Fire Tattvas). Science also binds time, space, and matter together through the theory of relativity. We can visibly see that death means we will no longer occupy space or be embodied in matter. The question that we then ask is: "Does time continue for us when we are no longer bound to space and matter?"

The scientist may say that when one comes to an end they all come to an end.

The mystics do not give us a direct answer because any answer they give us will be sifted through the history of the ahamkara. Instead they allude to something, enticing us to draw our attention closer and closer to the question, in order for us to be transformed enough to know the answer that is never spoken but is revealed in the silence of the "knowing" heart.

They ask that we look to all of these as the manifestation of a non-local event – infinity beyond time that the mind, with all its measuring and delineating, cannot begin to approach. But Prajna, that Knower of the heart that is so close to infinity, is able to understand.

The question is one of focus. If your point of focus is entirely on the "external," the body and personality, the triangles, circles, and hexagons of the yantra, then yes, the ancients would agree with the scientists that there is a transformation that can be called death. When you shift the focus to the internal which is eternal, the question is all that dies.

In *The Mandukya Upanishad*, which we have been glimpsing throughout this book, the word used to describe the body is Vaishvanara. This ancient perspective says that in order to form the atoms, molecules, and cells that make up the human body, a continuum of intention and activity took place: that was, each birth, be it of a human being or of the wave of a particle of an atom, required the active participation of the entire universe. According to this philosophy this universe was not an accident of chemical reactions but a creation with a purpose. Vaishvanara is not a single body, it is all bodies, manifesting an interconnectedness and interdependence – be it of the cells of an individual body or entire bodies that appear to be separated by time and space. Thus we are the daughters and sons of the universe, not merely individual children of individual parents.

When we see this possibility we participate in a vision of all life as one life. When we live as part of this universal oneness, we cease to wonder why the cells in the petri dish were alarmed by the death of nasal cells in the next room. When we live within the consciousness of Vaishvanara we directly experience the miracle of autopoiesis – the theory we encountered in the Fourth Wave of life as "self-making," in continuous re-creation of itself. Life always continues. But we will only know the nature of that life when we have let our attention be equally enraptured by the inner Prajna, the Knower.

In order for that to happen we will use our aging to clear our minds and our hearts through our practices. Only then will we replace the fear of death with a knowledge of life.

Ever-Decreasing Circles

We can sacrifice our lives for someone else, but we cannot die in place of another. Edna, whom you met in the first chapter, prayed for that as her daughter was dying: "I would have given anything to trade places with her. I just kept praying, 'Take me, please take me and let her live.'" But trading places is simply not possible.

Just as we begin to contemplate our own mortality, our loved ones – our parents, our partners, our friends – begin to die. We listen to their eulogies and we mourn their passing, slowly allowing ourselves to adjust to the death through the process of grieving. In just the last few decades medicine has come to acknowledge the enormous impact grief has on us. Some psychiatrists now believe that between 10 and 15 per cent of people who pass through mental health clinics are suffering from unresolved grief. In our sophisticated, technological world we have become so good at pushing back the barriers of death and, when that is no longer possible, hiding it behind banks of machinery and tubes and flashing lights, that we have become extremely bad at mourning.

Grieving is a pain that is almost unbearable – in the literal sense of the word. It is very often too much for us to bear on our own and we need the help of those around us to help contain and carry it.

Does the pain of grief ever go away? Are we ever reconciled to a beloved's death? Probably not, but we can bring to our own grieving and that of our friends what Ron Kurtz, founder of the Hakomi Method of psychotherapy, advised: "Sensitivity and time."[4]

We have to learn to offer each other more than simply a smile and our presence at the funeral of a loved one. We have to embrace grief as an essential part of our life's experience and be willing to allow it into our homes and our lives. After all, death is coming home again as more and more people are opting to die at home surrounded by those they love rather than in a hospital hooked up to monitors being watched by strangers. When death touches someone we know, we have to be open to their pain because it may be more than they can endure on their own.

Whatever our perspective on death, once we are the aging generation of our community, we have to begin to consider it. And we need to consider it in a sober and inquiring way rather than a morbid one. We have to

Turn and Face the Other Way.

This means even while we are enjoying the pleasure of life flowing through us, fulfilling our dreams, being open and in touch and prepared for the transformations that life demands of us, we have to know that our orientation has changed and we are headed not toward the beginning of this individual life but toward its end. And that surely must mean, first of all, an acknowledgment that we belong both to a moment and to eternity.

And while we contemplate this mystery, we can show our love and affection for the people around us by letting them know what we think of death and what personal arrangements we would like them to make for us when we die. Our aging generation must now lift the taboo off death, even as we lifted it off sex in the 1960s. We must talk about it – with people older than ourselves to learn from them, and with people younger than ourselves to both learn and teach.

We must train ourselves in self abandonment until we retain
nothing of our own.

MEISTER ECKHART[5]

Turning to face the other way means challenging the conditioning
of a lifetime that has led us to doubt the existence of anything that
connects us to each other, to the past or to the future. Riding this
wave means taking control of all of our life in a way that we are
wholly unaccustomed to – because it requires taking full responsibility for ourselves. As isolated individuals we are reduced, whatever the arena of our activities – social, political, etc. – to being cogs
in a wheel whose direction is determined by forces outside ourselves. Once we recognize ourselves as a part of the whole, inter-
connected with every other part, we become participants in
creation.

If the great mystics who sailed this sea ahead of us are correct,
the true order of creation is sacrificial: nothing exists for itself alone
and all things exist for the sake of another. Using this perspective,
sacrifice returns our life and death to the original meaning of that
word: making sacred. From the cell that dies so that others around
it may live to the breath we breathe in and out, life lives by sacrifice. The whole of creation is dependent upon our coming into
being, living, and dying – our presence here makes this creation
what it is and without us it would be something else entirely. We
are called upon to make our lives sacred by turning to that which is
immortal – the Unlimited – and paying it as much heed as we pay
to that which is momentary.

Like Abraham offering up his son in accordance with the
instructions of God, we too must offer up that into which we have
poured our creativity, the I-maker, doing this "until we retain nothing of our own."

Infinity, the Eternal, sacrifices itself to become the One bound by time and space. Death gives us the opportunity to offer our limitations back into the sacrifice in order to realize infinity. The I-maker and its tendency to look to that which furthers its own interests is seen as only a part of the whole rather than the whole itself. The focus of our practices now must be on abandoning the I-maker as our telescope on the world, and finding a much deeper, much wider perspective than it is able to offer. If we do this we have a chance of grasping all that it means to be human, all that is part of our "human ensemble."

> The whole sound Aum
> Is unbroken in its sounding –
> One indivisible word out of three divisible letters.
> As the whole Aum it is the fourth state –
> Beyond present, past and future,
> Beyond waking, dreaming and deep sleep.
> The Self is Aum, the Whole.
> One who knows this merges with the Self.

THE MANDUKYA UPANISHAD 12[6]

The three letters "A," "U," "M," which when pronounced together become the sound Aum, allow us an understanding of the "human ensemble." The letter "A" designates the body, Vaishvanara, "all bodies as one body." The letter "U" designates our cognitive faculties, the inner instrument, which the Upanishad calls Taijasa, "the Radiant Being." The letter "M" designates the awareness that is the portal to the Infinite and is called Prajna, "the Knower." These three letters only represent these different aspects of ourselves when they are sounded as one word – the long intonation of Aum done on the out-breath. And this is the final aspect of the self which the text calls Turiya, that which is beyond the other three and which they are part of. Time, space, and matter are bound together by their continuation. Like the sound of Aum being chanted, their togetherness cannot be scattered. Death may be a change in the pitch or tone, but in truth, nothing began and nothing ends.

When we live in this wholeness, death is not a stumbling into darkness, it is a part of the mystery of life still unfolding. Having taken full responsibility for ourselves, we walk boldly into the next big adventure, trusting the Self that brought us into creation to continue to reveal itself to us. Then we become the light that illuminates history rather than the tragedy in its pages.

There is only one Self
And it dwells within all beings –
Whole yet everywhere
It appears in this creation
In the same way that the moon reflects on dark water.

The life of this body
Is like a jar enclosing space.
When the jar shatters,
Only the jar shatters
And space remains whole and undifferentiated.

All bodies are like the jar:
Unceasingly forming and shattering.
And even though we may be unaware
That which is remains eternally the same.

THE BRAHMABINDU UPANISHAD VERSES 12, 13 AND 14[7]

We Are Sailing...

May we, O Waters,
Come to you for our nourishment and for our shelter.
Give to us that life-force
That you possess in such abundance.

RIG VEDA X.9

It was Rod Stewart who gave us the refrain that reminds us that we are sailing. The process of aging is new for us and navigating its waves requires our full consciousness and commitment. But once we have celebrated whichever birthday we consider takes us into "middle age," we are on the waters and we are indeed sailing.

We can continue to see growing old as a tragedy of life, as some horrible mistake of evolution. Or we can sing as we sail, knowing that this is the ocean that could take us to freedom. The choice of perspective is always our own – but we are on the ocean.

As we sail inexorably towards the horizon, the light of death shines beyond it, focusing our attention on the ultimate question: What is it that exists in that sacred space between knower and known that constructed them both and all the rest of creation?

> "Bend near to me!" he whispered in Govinda's ear. "Come still nearer ..."
>
> Although surprised, Govinda was compelled by a great love ... he leaned close to him and touched his forehead with his lips. As he did this something wonderful happened ... He no longer saw the face of his friend Siddhartha. Instead he saw other faces, many faces, a long series, a continuous stream of faces – hundreds, thousands, which all came and disappeared and yet all seemed to be there at the same time ...

HERMANN HESSE[8]

Chapter 12

Riding the Wave of
Turning to Face the Other Way

We have always been in awe of death. The monuments arising from
that awe, like the great pyramids of Egypt and the Taj Mahal of India, still
inspire us now, centuries after they were built. The 20th century perhaps
saw the most concerted withdrawal from the consciousness of death that
the human family has undergone in its history. The Victorians are usually
blamed for demanding that the bereaved bear their loss with a "stiff
upper lip." Yet all the evidence points to the Victorians encouraging
public displays of mourning with tears and grieving. Thus the modern
reticence about death probably has more to do with the advance of
science in the last century than with the influence of Victorian manners.

We split the atom and we put men on the moon, we probe Mars
and we replace entire organs in living people. Yet death still haunts
us, and if modern medicine with all its technology cannot defeat
death, it can send it to a private room and hide it behind banks of
bleeping machines and monitors with flashing lights. Technology
triumphs even as the person connected to it dies.

As science relegated death to the column of a problem still
to be solved, we lost touch with its mystery. But we are getting
in touch with it again. As already mentioned, more and more of
us are electing to die at home, surrounded by those we love. The

hospice movement, which gives patients a place to die in dignity being cared for by those they love, has grown enormously in the last 20 years. What remains is for us to draw the mystery of death closer to us and make it part of our journey into being fully human.

One of the most poignant burial stories I have ever encountered was not a modern one, but one from a past so ancient that no language existed to describe the scene for us. In *Origins* by Richard Leakey and Roger Lewin, the story of the "Shanidar man" unfolds.[1] In the Shanidar cave high in the Zagros mountains of Iraq, a Neanderthal man was buried by his community, his tribe, or family. Yarrow, cornflower, thistle, hyacinth, and other flowers were carefully placed around the body that was laid on a bed of woody horsetail. Even the Neanderthals, who had no verbal language, obviously had a keen self-awareness and sense of a human spirit. They were able to look at a horizon beyond the need for tools and the hunt, and pay tribute to one of their own who no longer walked with them. I think often of the family in that cave in the distant past of our own struggle towards being a self-aware humanity, walking out to pick the flowers that will adorn the burial site. And the prayer I often whisper is that we find a way of returning to that kind of grace.

As long as the fear of death or a vision of death as the ultimate failure binds us, we cannot live freely. While we live and give our full attention to living we have to turn our attention to the end of our life and be prepared to live, to really live, with the mystery of death. Living with that mystery means that we do not become bound by any system, but seek the freedom of movement towards the mystery.

The ancients used to bury tools and jewelry and money, and even food and slaves, with their dead, for the use of the departed. If part of the mystery of death is the probing of our survival, another part must be what survives? What is it we take with us when we leave this body?

A particularly wise old monk, Swami Krishnananda, whom I traveled to Rishikesh at the foothills of the Himalayas many times to listen to, addressed the question one day when I was tired and uncomfortable and fidgeting and wishing I was somewhere else. He pinned me down with his characteristic penetrating gaze and asked, "So, what is it that you think you will take with you into death?" The question was part of a reply to someone else, but as he asked it he looked so directly at me I knew I was meant to stay and hear the answer. There was a brief pause, then he continued, "Let me tell you, you will not take your wealth or your wife or your husband, you will not take your children or your position or your reputation. The only thing that you will take with you into death is what you think and what you feel."

What we think and what we feel. Do we even know what we are thinking and feeling at any given moment? The vast majority of our life is conducted in unconsciousness. Do we therefore know what we will be taking with us? Any given moment is the moment of death. And if Swami Krishnananda was right, at the moment of death our thoughts and feelings are what we take into eternity. The thought scared me into some kind of consciousness, some kind of wakefulness and self-awareness.

In addition to all the other kinds of self-knowledge that we have been practicing through the previous chapters we need urgently to examine all that we think and feel about death. The heart and mind need not only to change in order to live, they need to change in order to die.

What is Death?

The first thing to inquire into is what you think and feel about death. Just like sex, you will have grown up with family mythologies about death that you need to bring into the light of awareness. Did your family even talk about death, or was that subject taboo, considered too "morbid?" How was death handled in your family and how has this influenced the way you think about it? How was mourning dealt with in your family?

Experiment by seeing how easy or difficult it is to open a discussion about these things with the people around you, the people you love and are closest to. Do they welcome the discussion or do they try and change the subject as quickly as possible? You will be discovering not only what you think about death but what those around you think about it—often by what they do not say.

Ask yourself some hard questions:

- How do you mourn?

If anyone close to you has died, how did you mourn? How has the loss of that person shaped who you are now?

There is no right or wrong way to mourn. Some people can let it all hang out and weep openly, while those who are more private by nature grieve in private. Whatever way you mourn, you must begin to become aware of it as a process of healing.

The psychiatrist George Engels was one of the first to look at the very specific tasks of healing grief and pointed out that like all healing it is a process. First we have to become reconciled to the loss. Even when death occurs after a prolonged illness or in old age there is a sense of unreality about it. Gradually, with patience and sensitivity, we have to reconcile ourselves to the loved one's death. Next, while not everyone is going to experience loss with the same degree of pain, there is always some pain involved when a person or a pet that is close to you dies. A denial or refusal of that pain can lead to an

emotional crisis like depression or anxiety, or even physical symp-
toms like headaches and irritable bowel syndrome.

• How comfortable is it for you to be with a friend who is mourning?

Once you have begun to examine and talk about death you will
become a more comforting person to those who are in mourning, but
right now how comfortable are you? Do you offer them a distraction,
like tea or a night out, or are you able to be with them and support
their mourning? Being surrounded by people who become uncomfortable or embarrassed by expressions of grief can be just about
the most unhelpful thing someone in the midst of mourning can
encounter. Ask yourself how easy you find it to be with a friend who is
expressing their grieving. How many of your friends would be able to
support your own grieving with patience and sensitivity? Which
friends would they be, and which do you think would try and distract
you with another topic, a different activity?

The pain of grieving, our own and that of others, is also something
we have to be prepared to open up to and be touched by as we age.
Then, when we least feel like it, we are called upon once again to re-
create ourselves because adjusting to life without the person who has
died is part of the process of grieving. This task is impossible to
accomplish overnight. As time unfolds, all that that person meant in
your life will reveal itself to you, and with each revelation you will have
to re-create yourself to adjust for the loss. Losing a partner will mean
different things to different people – a close companion for some, the
household breadwinner for others. The loss of a parent will mean different things at different ages. Whatever the loss, the grieving person
has to become adjusted to a world in which they no longer have
direct contact with the other person.

When we are finally able to invest the emotions we felt for the person who has died in another, then we can be said to have healed. This
does not mean we have forgotten the other, but it does mean that we

who have been left among the living have been freed from pain and are able to love again. Do we still mourn? Of course we do, but we are not stuck, we are continually re-creating ourselves.

• How do you want to die?

If it is a matter of choice for you, when the time comes do you want to be at home or in a hospital? Whom would you like around you? Can you ask them now? How do they react when you discuss it? Very often the first thing someone will say when you broach the subject is something like "What's made you so morbid?" You will have to be prepared to laugh and explain that it is not morbidity but a step in taking responsibility for your life – which includes death.

Examining the answer to this question will also lead you to look at whether you want extraordinary measures taken on your behalf if you are not conscious. Again, there is no right or wrong here – you might well say to those around you that you want all measures possible taken to keep you alive, or you might well feel that after some limited measures you would like to be left to die. The point is that it is your decision – you are not leaving your own death to darkness and you are showing loving compassion for those you love by taking these decisions out of their hands. Ask yourself if you would like to make a living will to cover these eventualities. Ask those around you if they would prefer you to make a living will so that your wishes are clear.

Meditations for Death and Dying

Absorption Meditation

In this meditation you are going to visualize the re-absorption of your vitality – your *prana*, organized through the tattvas – into the cosmos, and then its re-emergence in you.

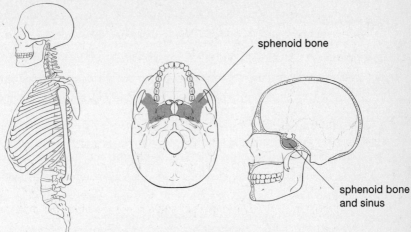

sphenoid bone

sphenoid bone
and sinus

The spine and sphenoid bone

Before you begin, look at the picture of the spine and sphenoid bone and visualize these in yourself so that the visualization exercises in the meditation are easier. The greatest meridian to the ancient Yogis was called Sushumna Nadi and it runs from the crown of the head down through the spine to the perineum (literally the place where your body meets the ground, between the anus and the genitalia). The "governing" chakra of all the chakras that relate directly to the body is Ajna Chakra, which is situated in the center of the head just above the sphenoid bone. In Japanese the sphenoid bone is known as Cho Kay Hotsu, "butterfly bone," and indeed this bone, with its four delicate wings, does somewhat resemble a butterfly. Once you have an internal vision of these you can proceed with the meditation.

I not only practice this meditation regularly myself, I often talk terminally ill patients, friends, or members of my community through it, as it is a kind of "practice" of the withdrawal of vitalities that happens at death. In Yoga this meditation is known as Laya, "Absorption."

• Sit or lie down in a way that allows the back, neck, and head to flow upward in their easy, undulating vertical line.

- Allow your weight to release down through the points of contact you have with the support beneath you.

- With each exhalation, as you release your weight downward, let any areas of tension dissolve, particularly the sockets of the eyes, the jaw, the throat, the abdomen, and the pelvis.

- Keep your awareness on your breath, feeling the cool air entering your nose, hitting the back of your throat and then warming as it descends into your lungs. As you breathe out, feel the warm air flowing up through your throat and leaving through your nose.

- Take your awareness to your spine and feel its roots deep in the pelvic basin. Follow the feeling right up your back, between the shoulder blades, up the back of the neck, right up into the skull, and then feel that its vitality continues up to the crown of the head.

- Visualize a radiant hollow tube running up your spine from its base to the crown of your head.

- As you breathe in, feel that a cool current flows down this tube, and as you breathe out, feel that a warm current rises up it. This is Sushumna Nadi, the Radiant Pathway, that stays open and connected to the rest of the universe. Prana is said to pour into it constantly and flow down it through the chakras, taking on the vibration of each tattva.

- Let the cool current that flows with the breath flow down to the base of the spine and continue right down to the perineum, to Muladhara Chakra that houses Earth Tattva.

- As you breathe out, let the warm current rising up Sushumna flow to the crown of the head, to Sahasrara, the thousand-petaled seat of the Divine, the opening through which your consciousness will flow when your body dies.

- Once you have done this several times, as the next cool current of the in-breath reaches Muladhara Chakra, feel that it picks up and absorbs the *prana* of earth, and as the warm current rises, feel it carry that earth vitality with it.

- On the next in-breath let the cool current reach the base of the spine to Svadhisthana Chakra, home to the vitality of water. Again feel the current gathering up the vitality of water, and as the warm current of the out-breath rises, let it carry up both earth and water.

- Let the next breath, the next cool current, reach Manipura Chakra, the home of fire vitality just behind the navel. Let the vitality be gathered up by the current, and as the warm current rises it will draw up earth, water, and fire.

- Then the cool current of the in-breath sinks into the chakra behind the heart, Anahata Chakra, and gathers up the vitality of wind, and the warm current rising on the out-breath carries up with it earth, water, fire, and wind.

- As the next cool current descends on the in-breath it reaches Vishuddha Chakra at the base of the throat and picks up the vitality of space, to be carried upward by the warm current of the out-breath with earth, water, fire, and wind.

- Focus entirely now on the out-breath and let earth, water, fire, wind, and space ascend and come to rest at the mystical area at the sphenoid bone. Feel as if these tattvas are all resting on that bone and that you are withdrawing your awareness from the body to that area. Hold that awareness for a few breaths, continually allowing your consciousness to be drawn into a sharp point of focus at this sacred space.

- Breathe in deeply, and as you breathe out slowly feel that warm current lift the tattvas and your consciousness up to the crown of your head.

- Feel the tattvas and your own individual consciousness all being gathered up by the larger forces of the universe, enfolded into the universal embrace as you let go ... let go.

- For as long as you can, hold this sense of having moved from being a local phenomenon bound by time and space to being a universal one.

- Then feel this cool current beginning to flow in through the crown of your head and down the center of your spine, down Sushumna Nadi. With each inhalation feel its force grow stronger and stronger.

- On the next in-breath feel that the force entering through the crown of your head brings with it Space Tattva and that it takes up its residence in Sushumna Nadi at the base of your neck.

- As you breathe out and feel the warm current rising, feel also Space Tattva reconnecting to you and sending its gifts of self-organization to all the systems, all the organs, and even the cells of your body.

- With the next in-breath Wind Tattva rushes in and quickly settles in Sushumna Nadi behind the heart.

- As you breathe out, feel its lightning-fast connections sending its gifts of movement and power throughout your body.

- Let the next in-breath bring fire and place it in Sushumna Nadi just behind the navel. As you breathe out and Fire Tattva reconnects to you, feel its warmth and its gifts of vision and transformation fill you.

- On the next in-breath let Water Tattva flow in with the vitality and be carried to its place at the base of the spine. As you breathe out, feel it making its connections to you and offering its gifts of creativity and deep ancestral memory.

- As you breathe in, feel this force bring with it Earth Tattva and carry it down to the perineum, where it gently returns it to its seat in you. As you breathe out, feel that Earth Tattva making deep connections within you, bringing you powers of stability and cohesion.

- As all of these tattvas resettle and reconnect with you, allow your sense of I to surrender to them and to their purpose.

- Remain in this consciousness for a few breaths before moving again.

All Breaths in One Breath

One of the quickest ways of breaking away from the lineage of violence we have been committed to and that is killing too many of us and depriving us of the gift of aging is to gain a true understanding of what it means to breathe.

Every time we breathe in, we breathe in approximately 10^{20} molecules – that's billions and billions of molecules. And each time we breathe out, we breathe out 10^{20} molecules. Not all that we are breathing in is made up of atmospheric gases. We are also breathing in atomic particles that other living beings have been breathing out into the atmosphere since life began. Our breath comes to us from a vast distance, from oceans and continents away. But it also comes to us from the vastness of time. The atmosphere that we live in is the same atmosphere that has been hugging the Earth since life began and an atmosphere was formed. So with each breath we breathe in the past, absorbing the molecules of all those who have lived on this planet before us. And when we breathe out, we breathe out billions of atomic particles of ourselves, and these particles will stay on the surface of our planet and be carried around in its atmosphere by its winds until this atmosphere ends.

Thus with each breath we are connecting to everything else on the planet. We do not know where each breath comes from, what great distances it has traveled to reach us; nor do we know where our breath and the parts of ourselves that we have breathed out will travel to. So we also connect to the past and the future.

Maintain this consciousness during the next meditation, which is best done at night just before going to sleep.

All Breaths in One Breath Meditation

- As you breathe in, feel that you are breathing in from a great distance away – from rainforests, oceans, and continents away your in-breath has come to you. And it brings with it the deepest past of life on our planet. Feel that through this inhalation you are connecting to that distance in space and time.
- As you breathe out, feel that your breath is picked up by unfelt winds and carried away from you to nourish rainforests, oceans, and continents far away. Feel also that you breathe into the future, as all that you have breathed out remains forever present.
- Keep this visualization going through several breaths, connecting yourself to the past and the future.

Healing the Original Wound

Take just a few moments to close your eyes and observe your body. Feel its contact with whatever is supporting it and with your skin, and feel its movement as you breathe. Become aware also of your breath, feeling the air entering and leaving you, and then the next wave of air being drawn into the stillpoint between breaths.

Next let yourself become aware of the thoughts drifting

through your consciousness – sometimes dense and impenetrable, sometimes quick, sometimes slow. Do not let your awareness drift off into the stream of thought, simply watch it.

You are aware of the body, aware of the breath, and even aware of the thoughts flowing in front of your consciousness, and you are that which is observing all of these. We are that which is observing and that which is observed. Somehow there is a fracture between these two realities. Healing this schism is the ultimate healing we bring to ourselves and to our world. As long as we ourselves are "two," we cannot possibly comprehend our oneness with all of creation. We engage in conflict because there is a perceived division. When we heal the wound of our own internal division, no division exists anywhere.

There is no one technique for this healing. It is all the techniques that you have been doing that bring you to a clearer understanding of where you are and what your relationship is with the rest of humanity. It is entering into a state of choiceless awareness. There is no observer to choose this or that. There is no this or that – there is only pure awareness. In that awareness observer and observed dissolve in a sacred Present.

This is the state of Turiya, beyond the boundaries of all that we know now and yet encompassing them. Prajna, the Knowing Self of the heart, Taijasa, the inner state of knowledge, and Vaishvanara, the body through which these contact the world, are enfolded by that pure awareness and are not experienced as "other."

In that state we live in non-violence. In that state we enjoy the beauty of the sunset without seeking to replicate and market the experience. In that awareness we inhale the perfume of the flower without crushing the life out of its petals to make a perfume to "own" its scent. In that choiceless awareness we are entirely reborn.

Is it possible Life saw that this was not the task of youth, with all its urgent demands, and now calls us into aging, when all youth's demands can be set aside, so that we can undertake the healing of this primal wound that keeps us all apart?

Thought creates a million images out of the ideal of Oneness. Awakened awareness – the buddhahood that we are all born to – moves us into the sacred space of Oneness.

Then, like all our teachers, we have to leave this gift for those who come after us.

Therefore, we do not give up.
Even as the man we are outside is wasting away
The man we are inside is being renewed from day to day.

2 CORINTHIANS 4:16

Bibliography

Daniel G. Amen, MD, *Change Your Brain, Change Your Life*, Times Books, 1998

John D. Barrow, *The Book of Nothing*, Vintage, 2000

Richard W. Boerstler and Hulen S. Kornfeld, *Life to Death: Harmonising the Transition*, Healing Arts Press, 1996

David Bohm and David Peat, *Science, Order and Creativity*, Routledge, 1987

J. Bronowski, *The Ascent of Man*, Book Club Associates, 1973

Deepak Chopra, *Ageless Body, Timeless Mind*, Rider, 1993

Paul Davies, *God and the New Physics*, Penguin Books, 1984

Paul Davies and John Gribbin, *The Matter Myth: Towards 21st Century Science*, Viking, 1992

Phyllis K. Davis, *The Power of Touch*, Hay House, Inc., 1999

David W. Deamer and Gail R. Fleischaker, *Origins of Life: The Central Concepts*, Jones and Bartlett Publishers, London, 1994

Thomas Hanna, *Somatics*, Addison Wesley, 1988

Linda Hartley, *Wisdom of the Body Moving: An Introduction to Body-Mind Centering*, North Atlantic Books, California, 1995

Herman Hesse, *Siddhartha*, Picador, 1998

Deane Juhan, *Job's Body: A Handbook for Bodywork*, Station Hill Press, 1989

Arthur Koestler, *The Ghost in the Machine*, Arkana, 1989

Swami Krishnananda, *Resurgent Culture*, The Divine Life Society, PO
    Shivanandanagar Dist., Tehri-Garhwal, UP, India

Ron Kurtz, *Body-Centered Psychotherapy: The Hakomi Method*,
    LifeRhythm, 1990

Richard Leakey and Roger Lewin, *Origins*, E. P. Dutton, New York, 1977

Lynne McTaggart, *The Field: The Quest for the Secret Force of the Universe*,
    HarperCollins, 2001

Meister Eckhart: *Selected Writings*, ed. Oliver Davies, Penguin Classics,
    1994

Thomas Merton, *The Collected Poems*, New York New Directions, 1977

Hugh Milne, *The Heart of Listening*, North Atlantic Books, Berkeley,
    California, 1998

Sherwin B. Nuland, *How We Die*, Vintage, 1997

Dr Dean Ornish, *Love and Survival*, Vermilion, 2001

Robert Ornstein and David Sobel, *The Healing Brain*, M. Papermac, 1989

Panchadasi, trans. Hari Prasad Shastri, Shanti Sadan, London

Candace Pert, PhD, *Molecules of Emotion*, Simon and Schuster, 1998

Maurice Merleau-Ponty, *Phenomonology of Perception*, trans. Colin Smith,
    Routledge, 2002

John Robbins, *Diet for a New America*, H. J. Kramer Books, California, and
    New World Library, 1998

Peter Tomkins and Christopher Bird, *The Secret Life of Plants*, Arkana,
    London, 1991

Chögyam Trungpa, *Cutting through Spiritual Materialism*, Shambhala
    Publications, 1987

Swami Venkatesananda, *Vasistha's Yoga*, SUNY

Swami Venkatesananda, *Multiple Reflections*, Chiltern Yoga Trust, San
    Francisco

Lyall Watson, *The Romeo Error*, Hodder & Stoughton, 1974

References

Chapter 1

1. Tom Kirkwood, *The Reith Lectures*, broadcast on BBC Radio 4, April 4th 2001
2. Swami Krishnananda, *Resurgent Culture*, The Divine Life Society, PO Shivanandanagar Dist., Tehri-Garhwal, UP, India
3. *The Chandogya Upanishad*, trans. Swami Ambikananda, unpublished
4. *The Uddhava Gita*, trans. Swami Ambikananda Saraswati, Frances Lincoln Ltd, 1999
5. *The Chandogya Upanishad*, op. cit.
6. *The Brhadaranyaka Upanishad*, trans. Swami Ambikananda, unpublished
7. Kirkwood, op. cit.

Chapter 2

1. *The Bhagavad Gita*, trans. Swami Ambikananda Saraswati, unpublished
2. Lynne McTaggart, *The Field: The Quest for the Secret Force of the Universe*, HarperCollins, 2001
3. Robert Ornstein and David Sobel, *The Healing Brain*, M. Papermac, 1989
4. Lyall Watson, *The Romeo Error*, Hodder & Stoughton, 1974
5. Thomas Merton, *The Collected Poems*, New York New Directions, 1977

Chapter 3

1. Arthur Koestler, *The Ghost in the Machine*, Arkana, 1989

Chapter 5

1. *The Chandogya Upanishad*, trans. Swami Ambikananda Saraswati, unpublished
2. Richard Leakey and Roger Lewin, *Origins*, E. P. Dutton, New York, 1977
3. J. Bronowski, *The Ascent of Man*, Book Club Associates, 1973
4. Candace Pert, PhD, *Molecules of Emotion*, Simon and Schuster, 1998
5. Chögyam Trungpa, *Cutting through Spiritual Materialism*, Shambhala Publications, 1987
6. Dr Dean Ornish, *Love and Survival*, Vermilion, 2001

Chapter 6

1. *The Narada Bhakti Sutras*, trans. Swami Ambikananda Saraswati, unpublished
2. Daniel G. Amen, MD, *Change Your Brain, Change Your Life*, Times Books, 1998
3. Deepak Chopra, *Ageless Body, Timeless Mind*, Rider, 1993
4. John Robbins, *Diet for a New America*, H. J. Kramer Books, California, and New World Library, 1998

Chapter 7

1. Phyllis K. Davis, *The Power of Touch*, Hay House, Inc., 1999
2. Deane Juhan, *Job's Body: A Handbook for Bodywork*, Station Hill Press, 1989
3. Sherwin B. Nuland, *How We Die*, Vintage, 1997
4. Thomas Hanna, *Somatics*, Addison Wesley, 1988

Chapter 8

1. Linda Hartley, *Wisdom of the Body Moving: An Introduction to Body-Mind Centering*, North Atlantic Books, California, 1995
2. Maurice Merleau-Ponty, *Phenomonology of Perception*, trans. Colin Smith, Routledge, 2002

Chapter 9

1. Swami Venkatesananda, personal correspondence
2. *The Brhadaranyaka Upanishad*, trans. Swami Ambikananda Saraswati, unpublished
3. Ibid.
4. David Bohm and David Peat, *Science, Order and Creativity*, Routledge, 1987
5. Swami Venkatesananda, *Multiple Reflections*, Chiltern Yoga Trust, San Francisco
6. *The Katha Upanishad*, trans. Swami Ambikananda Saraswati, Frances Lincoln Ltd, 2000

Chapter 10

1. Swami Venkatesananda, *Vasistha's Yoga*, SUNY
2. Paul Davies and John Gribbin, *The Matter Myth: Towards 21st Century Science*, Viking, 1992
3. *The Taittiriya Upanishad*, trans. Swami Ambikananda, unpublished

Chapter 11

1. *The Uddhava Gita*, trans. Swami Ambikananda, Frances Lincoln Ltd, 1999
2. Richard W. Boerstler and Hulen S. Kornfeld, *Life to Death: Harmonising the Transition*, Healing Arts Press, 1996
3. *The Mandukya Upanishad*, trans. Swami Ambikananda, unpublished
4. Ron Kurtz, *Body-Centered Psychotherapy: The Hakomi Method*, LifeRhythm, 1990
5. Meister Eckhart: *Selected Writings*, ed. Oliver Davies, Penguin Classics, 1994
6. *The Mandukya Upanishad*, op. cit.
7. *The Brahmabindu Upanishad*, trans. Swami Ambikananda, unpublished.
8. Herman Hesse, *Siddhartha*, Picador, 1998

Chapter 12
1. Richard E. Leakey and Roger Lewin, *Origins*, E. P. Dutton, New York, 1977

Index

Make
www.thorsonselement.com
your online sanctuary

Get online information, inspiration and
guidance to help you on the path to physical
and spiritual well-being. Drawing on the integrity
and vision of our authors and titles, and with
health advice, articles, astrology, tarot, a
meditation zone, author interviews and events
listings, www.thorsonselement.com is a great
alternative to help create space and peace
in our lives.

So if you've always wondered about practising
yoga, following an allergy-free diet, using the
tarot or getting a life coach, we can point you
in the right direction.

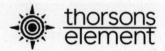

thorsons
element